Navigating the Road of Infertility

Navigating the Road
of Infertility

Chrissie Lee Kahan and Aaron Michael Kahan

ISBN-13: 9780997933307
ISBN-10: 0997933305
Library of Congress Control Number: 2016913245
King Kahan Publishing, LLC, Parkville, MD

To those of you who have been forced to travel down this road. Your strength, courage, and hope are more inspiring than you may realize. We dedicate this book to you!

Prologue

June 2016

WE FLED TO THE OCEAN, the one place that gives us respite when we are in dire need. While there, we reflected on how great it was that we could be shepherds of two souls so bereft of love and care. And we mourned in a way that was so selfish and yet so giving. We wanted nothing but the best of life for these two little ones of whom we were told, "Yes, they are yours, but no, they are not."

This was supposedly implied by the great Department of Social Services. It was to have been an unspoken agreement upon the girls' arrival. They saw us as a lovely middle-class couple who would simply shut up and take the check. We still aren't quite sure where this assumption originated from, given our prerequisite position of "preadoptive resource only." Chrissie and I learned that this position does not truly exist. There are merely compliant and noncompliant, and we were definitely the latter of the two in their eyes.

While lying in isolation, on a beach drenched in fog and rain and seasonal, mild cold, we thought. We thought about how this situation was better. How it might actually be worse. Chrissie and I sat on a damp balcony overlooking a gray ocean and an even grayer sky that very much mimicked and almost mocked our mental state.

We didn't know how to feel. We didn't know where to be. We didn't know what to do. We only knew that these poor girls who should have been ours were ours no longer. These girls could have been in the care of their heroin-addict mother, who wanted nothing from them but government money. We also knew this was something that we couldn't abide, but it was made painfully clear that we had no control over it.

During our time there on the great gray beaches of Ocean City, we decided that we were going to start our own family. We decided that fate and our previous trials could take a long walk off the short pier. Somehow, some-way, we were going to have a kid! It was a reaffirmed determination, one that we had lost sight of in our hopes of fostering to adopt.

CHAPTER 1

The Red-Brick Road

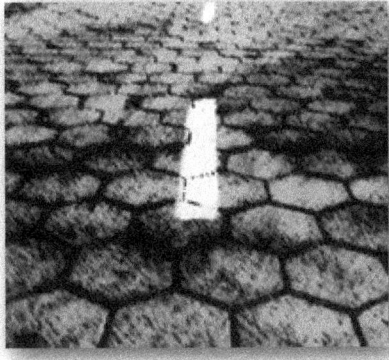

February 2012

EXCITED, DETERMINED, HOPEFUL, DISAPPOINTED, FRUSTRATED, sad, shocked, and numb—this is the cycle of emotions each couple goes through every month without conception. Every doctor appointment, procedure, and let-down, this is the emotional cycle that would repeat. Each couple who is forced off the highway of planned pregnancy to be shoved onto the lonely exit ramp to infertility road sadly knows this cycle all too well.

Our road started less than a year after we were married. We never could have prepared for the twists and turns our life and marriage were about to take.

It all started simply enough. On a romantic weekend getaway, we started talking about how amazing it would be to create a little version of the two of us. So of course, after hours of picturing the different characteristics of each of us our baby would have, the birth control was thrown out, and we were on our way to getting pregnant. We even joked about how easily it would happen, because of course we were still in the "honeymoon period" and couldn't keep our hands off each other.

As we shared our excitement with others, purposefully along with accidentally (being the planner I was, I had downloaded an ovulation app and aligned the matching ovulation calendar to my shared work calendar with my office), we were told not to talk about it, as we would jinx ourselves. Being the open person I was, I didn't understand trying to hide the prospect of such an exciting new journey in my life.

But sadly, the joke started to be on us as month after month passed with no sign of pregnancy. And I started to feel the pressure of people wondering why I was not yet pregnant. Each month, I would get excited when my period didn't come, wondering if this was it, tricking my mind into believing we were pregnant. Some months it even felt as though my body was pregnant, as it was expressing the hopeful thoughts in my mind and manifesting pregnancy symptoms that I of course had read about on the Internet.

Then, at the first sign of blood, I would feel my heart sink in my chest, defeated, like I wasn't trying hard enough. Each period was another red brick leading me further down infertility road.

CHAPTER 2

The What's Wrong Cyclone

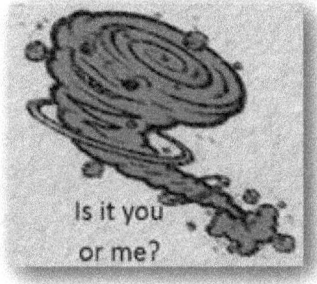

Is it you or me?

I HAVE BEEN WITH MY gynecologist since I was sixteen. I have always trusted her opinion and valued her input, especially because I tend to be a hypochondriac who comes prepared to each visit with a multitude of questions. So when I asked her if I should be concerned that we hadn't become pregnant after over six months of trying, I believed her when she assured me that everyone's body is different, that I was healthy, and that I should give it more time. Of course, I had researched causes of not getting pregnant on WebMD, and I went through my list: Should I lose weight? Should I eat only organic? Should we stop drinking completely? Was my husband affected due to the years he had spent with his laptop on his lap? Were we doing it too much or not enough? Again, she reiterated that everyone was different and told me not to be too concerned or put pressure on myself, but to just give it more time.

So we continued to try to conceive, each month utilizing the ovulation app and the ovulation kits available over the counter. I even started putting my legs up in the air for a timed amount after intercourse. Talk about taking the romance and fun out of sex! There is nothing like, "Honey, the pink pad says I'm ovulating; we only have a set period of time. Let's do it as much as we can." With all these measures in place and the overwhelming pressure with the lack of results, it wasn't long before Aaron and I were fighting. And there is nothing like fighting to diminish your sex drive.

It felt like my body was betraying me. I am a planner. I'm used to having a goal with an allotted time frame, putting in the hard work, and utilizing resources to achieve the goal. I didn't understand why something that was supposed to be so natural and came so easily for most people was such a daunting task for me. I say it comes easily to most people, not to offend those who deal with infertility, but because as you are experiencing trials of infertility, you literally feel like everyone around you is becoming pregnant.

Aaron and I started to play the blame game. Quietly at first, in our own minds, secretly wondering what was wrong and whose fault it was. Then, out loud. Because of course I continued to read the articles on the Internet regarding infertility causes, and I needed a way to fix what I thought was the issue. So Aaron's lack of taking vitamins or the alcoholic drinks he enjoyed became the reason in my mind. It then felt like I was working to try to fix things, and he was not taking it as seriously.

Since he is six years younger, it did not seem like he felt the same pressure about time constraints that I did. It had taken me to the age of thirty-one to marry him, my soul mate and the love of my life. At thirty-two, I felt like I was really running out of time to have a family.

My good friend at the time who was hearing my ongoing fertility struggle shared her story about how it took her six years to conceive. She explained that she had to get a sonogram to determine that something was going on internally that needed to be corrected, and she was the one who convinced me that I needed to do the same.

It was a year after we had started trying to have a baby when I had my yearly checkup. Coincidentally, Aaron, who also saw my doctor as his primary physician, had his appointment directly after mine. I shared my frustration at the lack of conception, and after my doctor went through her usual advice of how it took time and I was healthy, I finally convinced her to order the sonogram. In examining Aaron, she took one look at his private area, specifically his pair of prime baby-making possessions, and told him he had varicocele. She recommended the name of a urologist for him to see.

Oh, varicocele! When I first heard the name, I pronounced it "variococelle" like it was an Italian pasta dish. So off to Google we went: "Varicocele: an enlargement of the veins within the scrotum." They often produce no symptoms but can cause low sperm production and decreased sperm quality, leading to infertility.

Bingo! We had found the cause, right? The reason we had struggled for over a year to conceive. Surely, this was it, and it could be corrected. We would just go to the urologist, get them removed, and then be able to get pregnant. I had no idea of the twists that were coming as we moved further down the infertility road.

Then, I took the turn for my sonogram appointment. Setting it up was easy enough, and it was only a couple of miles from my work. "Come with a full bladder," they said. Everyone I talked to shared that it was no big deal. So I gulped down my two liters of water and anxiously waited in the waiting room. After twenty minutes of feeling like my bladder was going to burst, I prompted the nurse behind the desk, who did not seem to understand the difficulty I was experiencing. Nevertheless, with an attitude, she sped up the process, and I was soon in the gown, with gel on, getting my first sonogram. The technician was very sweet and listened to my story. She shared some of her own of the patients who came in. This put me more at ease. She told me that she couldn't see anything and that I looked completely healthy. She also shared that she couldn't wait to see me back there when I was pregnant to get a sonogram of my baby.

Driving straight to work after this process, I had mixed feelings. I was supposed to feel good, right? Nothing was wrong, and I looked healthy. My secretary immediately told me that she knew I was healthy and nothing was wrong, along with several other people close to me. Was this response supposed to make me feel better? If there was nothing wrong with me, then why was this taking so long? Why did I feel so inadequate, and why was there this sinking feeling inside me? Well, the good thing about being an assistant principal in an elementary school is that you don't have too long to ponder anything before being thrown into the tasks or issues of the day, so these thoughts were fleeting.

It wasn't until two weeks later, when Aaron and I were driving to his sister's graduation in South Carolina, that I heard from my doctor's technician. "Hi, Mrs. Kahan. We got the results of your sonogram, and they found a benign uterine fibroid tumor. These are very common in women. Most times, these tumors do not have a detrimental impact. They can, however, cause infertility depending on their location." Once I regained my breathing and composure after hearing the word *tumor*, I asked when I could get it taken out. I didn't even have Google or WebMD open, but I knew that this foreign mass needed to come out of me. "Oh, our office does not do that procedure. You will have to contact a specialist. You can go through your insurance." Uh, never had to do that before. Thankfully, it was a nine-hour drive, which gave me the opportunity to get our insurance provider on the phone. It wasn't long before I had a referral to a fertility center with a highly praised fertility specialist. I was going to get this taken care of. This was surely something that could be fixed. But there was this foreign object growing inside me. Yikes, could this be causing more damage to my health than just infertility? To the trusty Internet.

From Healthline.com:

> What are Fibroids? Fibroids are abnormal growths that develop in or on a woman's uterus. It is unclear why fibroids develop, but several factors may influence their formation, such as hormones and family history. About 70 to 80 percent of women experience fibroids by the age of 50. Sometimes, these tumors become quite large and cause severe abdominal pain and heavy periods. In other cases, they cause no signs or symptoms at all.

Hmm, what were the chances that my fibroid tumor was causing no signs or symptoms and was small? Thinking about my life thus far and the difficult road we were on in trying to conceive, I was not real optimistic. So, I continued to the symptoms:

Your symptoms will depend on the location and size of the tumor(s) and how many tumors you have.

Symptoms of fibroids may include:

- heavy bleeding between or during your periods
- pain in the pelvis and/or lower back
- increased menstrual cramping
- increased urination
- pain during intercourse
- menstruation that lasts longer than usual
- pressure or fullness in your lower abdomen
- swelling or enlargement of the abdomen

As I read through the list, I said to myself, "Check, check, check, check, check, check, check." It all made sense as to why I felt like my body was changing and I wasn't in control. I had thought maybe the process of conceiving was decreasing my sex drive and enthusiasm to be with my husband romantically, but now it made more sense. The periods with the heavy flow and cramping that lasted for seven to ten days could all be explained. I read on to the treatment options, which listed medications, surgery, and minimally invasive procedures. I just knew in my heart it would end up having to be surgically removed. However, it was well out of my control at this point, so I was off to meet with the specialist.

CHAPTER 3

We're Off to See the Fertility Wizard

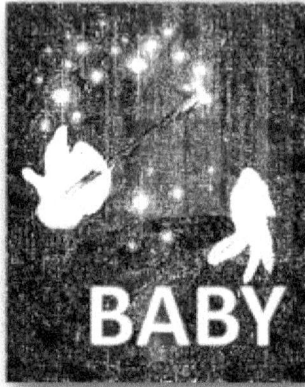

June 2014

I'M A VERY SEQUENTIAL PERSON. So after the initial shock of realizing there was a foreign thing growing inside me, I immediately started focusing on the steps I needed to take to get the tumor removed. It made sense now why I had been struggling with my health and my libido. Most people think a female doesn't have the same type of sex drive as a man. However, I had been blessed my whole life with a very high sex drive. I could have fifteen orgasms from intercourse alone. This was something that my female friends did not understand, as their bodies were not the same as mine. But I had enjoyed having this ability for my whole life, up until the past several months. Sex was painful, I wasn't as lubricated, and I got my first-ever yeast infection. I had assumed it was just the stress of not being able to conceive that was causing these changes, but the fact that it could all be caused by a tumor that I could have taken out of me seemed like a relief. So I focused on the steps I needed to take action to get it removed. The first step was to meet with the specialist.

Soon, my appointment was scheduled, and Aaron and I nervously drove to meet with a fertility specialist. I had read the reviews about her online, which were very good. As we drove up, I realized the office was centered one block from my high school and college apartment. I took this as a good sign and reflected back to my happy, carefree times to divert my mind from the anxiety I felt walking into the center.

Walking in, I couldn't help but notice all the couples sitting in the waiting room. You could feel the emotions coming off them—the sadness of being in that position, but also the relentless hope that this was going to be the place that helped them get the miracle of life they had been craving, unable to achieve on their own.

After filling out the appropriate paperwork, we of course had to pay a fee of thirty dollars just for seeing the specialist. Thirty dollars every time we needed to come to this office was not something I had thought of. But it was necessary. After all, what wouldn't you be willing to pay to get your health back and the chance to have one of your dreams come true, right?

We were taken back to see the specialist quite quickly. Not the normal standard procedure of when you go to your doctor for your scheduled appointment and then have to wait another thirty minutes until you are able to get seen. Hey, if that thirty-dollar fee gets you back quicker, it's well worth it. I just tried to think of it as a kind of VIP service except for fertility and not as fun as getting into a club in Vegas—which, as I was walking back, was one of the places I was wishing I was in. Any other place, in any other situation that focused on fun and happiness instead of a lack of conception and uterine fibroid tumors. Ugh, just thinking the name of it made me want to get that thing out of my body immediately.

When my fertility specialist walked in, she of course was not what I pictured. Very matter-of-fact and to-the-point kind, but not warm and fuzzy. So I went through our story and proceeded to ask when my tumor could be removed. She quickly backed me up several steps by going through the process of procedures that needed to occur before we even talked about the potential of surgery. Invasive surgery was a last step that depended on the size and location of the tumor. She said a lot of other, more medical things, but my mind tuned out. Thankfully, Aaron was listening. His father having been an ER doctor and his mom a nurse, I knew I could count on him to relay in normal human terms the explanation of the processes we were receiving. I tuned in just in time to hear steps—thank God, something I could wrap my brain around. "Call this number to schedule your HSG (hysterosalpingogram). You will have to do this at the hospital with this doctor. Then, you will schedule your water HSG at our office. After that, we'll determine the next course of action, as we will have a better indication of the size and location of your tumor." Check, check, and go. I still wasn't sure if I liked my specialist or not. She didn't seem to understand that I was matter-of-fact just like her, and I knew my body. This thing was hurting me and needed to come out. But of course, like everything else, it would have to be a process.

To the next part, the HSG. This was a procedure I probably should have spent more time googling on the Internet. My first thought was, *MSG like in Chinese food?* No. My next thought was, *Oh my God, I have to go to the hospital for this. Yikes.* I guess that's why I didn't do more research. After I had to go through the intricate process of scheduling the procedure, making sure my insurance would cover it, and making sure it was only on the day/times specific medical staff would be there, I was exhausted. Not to mention that hospitals were not my favorite places after my stepdad had died in one just two years ago. But at least this procedure would be in the hospital I was born in, the hospital that saved my life as a miracle premature baby. That had to be a good sign, right? Anyway, the HSG. Before I get into technical terms, let me just say that this is a procedure that military personnel, evil villains, or anyone else you can think of who could possibly torture someone to get information should use. Forget waterboarding, prying off people's fingernails, and even that scene in the movie *Taken* where Liam Neeson has the kidnapper attached to the short-circuited power line, giving him jolt after jolt. The HSG tops all of that, especially when you have a rapidly growing tumor inside you.

Looking back, it's a good thing I didn't know what I was encountering, or I'm not sure I would have gone through with it.

Technically, according to AdvancedFertility.com, an HSG is a "fertility test for tubal patency and normalcy of the uterine cavity."

> A hysterosalpingogram, or HSG is an important test of female fertility potential. The HSG test is a radiology procedure usually done in the radiology department of the hospital. Radiographic contrast (dye) is injected into the uterine cavity through the vagina and cervix. The uterine cavity fills with dye, and if the fallopian tubes are open, dye fills the tubes and spills into the abdominal cavity. This shows whether the fallopian tubes are open or blocked, and whether a blockage is at the junction of the tube and uterus or at the other end. Other things that can be seen on a HSG include that the uterine cavity is evaluated for the presence of fibroid tumors.

On to the actual procedure. Again, I was thankful for the business of my job, as it did not allow too much thinking time. So on the day of this procedure, I hustled from work and navigated the long hallways of the hospital until I found the radiology department. I always tend to wonder to myself when I'm in hospitals if it is at all like what is portrayed on the popular show *Grey's Anatomy*. Focusing on the doctors, nurses, and other personnel and attempting to align them to the show seemed to pass the anxiety in my mind. After hearing some awkward insurance conversations, it was my turn to sign in. Form after form, and polite small talk ensued as I walked back to the waiting area. I couldn't help but notice the patients who were battling cancer along my way, so I said a prayer for them internally. The focus on the people, although it provided a good distraction, did not take away my anxiety. So to Candy Crush it was, my favorite distraction when I needed a quick escape from life. It wasn't long before Aaron and then my mom met me in the waiting room. Most people would think that it was overdramatic for them to be there, but they loved me, were concerned, and wanted to show their support. Of course for me, that's always difficult, because I tend to be the strong one in my relationships. So instead of focusing on my nervousness and anxiety, I had to put on a brave face. When my name was called, it felt like a long, foreign walk down a very cold hallway. The technician who walked me was explicit in the instructions for the disrobing, the protocol of putting clothes in the bag, and so on. The environment was so sterile—cold—overwhelming.

Now for the actual procedure. Again, I turn to AdvancedFertility.com prior to getting into my own explanation.

The woman lies on the table on her back and brings her feet up into a "frog leg" position. The doctor places a speculum in the vagina and visualizes the cervix. Either a soft, thin catheter is placed through the cervical opening into the uterine cavity or an instrument called a tenaculum is placed on the cervix and then a narrow metal cannula is inserted through the cervical opening. Contrast is slowly injected through the cannula or catheter into the uterine cavity. An x-ray picture is taken as the uterine cavity is filling and then additional contrast is injected so that the tubes should fill and begin to spill into the abdominal cavity. More x-ray pictures are taken as this "fill and spill" occurs. When both tubes spill dye, the woman is often asked to roll to one side or the other slightly to give a slightly oblique x-ray image which can further delineate the anatomy.

Sounds lovely, right? Ugh, yuck, I just kept telling myself that I was going through this so I could be healthy again. Of course, with my outgoing personality, it has never been a problem to make small talk with doctors and nurses, even when I am naked in a gown that hardly covers anything, with my private area exposed for all in the room to see. It wasn't long until I shared the story of how I got there. The radiologist was very good; he accurately described what he would be doing throughout all stages of the process. Even though it was excruciatingly uncomfortable, I am logical and sequential, so I found comfort in knowing the steps. But when it got to the part where I was told to lie on my side, I felt like Ross in the show *Friends* when he had that weird growth, and doctor after doctor was being called in to try to diagnose it. I heard one of the four or five medical professionals say, "Oh, wow!"

Silly faith filled me; I thought God had removed the tumor from my uterus and shouted out hopefully, "Is it gone?" A long pause ensued as I heard the medical professionals tell me no and then ask me to continue to turn so they could get a better view. *Sure, I'll completely turn on my stomach with a catheter stuck inside me so you can get a better view? No problem, not uncomfortable at all.* As they continued to marvel at the view of my tumor, I waited on the edge of the cold, gray hospital table. A tumor the size of a grapefruit, growing to the size of a coconut, was taking up residence in a large portion of my uterus. It was in a very interesting place, apparently, that was uncommon for fibroid tumors. Oh, good; now what?

Since all medical professionals like to be thorough, the regular HSG was not enough. Two days later, being the efficient planner that I was, I had my water HSG appointment. This time at the fertility center. Sadly, my specialist was on vacation, so her partner was the one who would be administering the test. When scheduling, I hadn't thought it to be a big deal, but I had no idea the kind of pain I would feel. The other fun factor in this was that, during the summer, there are three people who run the school's office: me, my principal, and my secretary. I was the only one scheduled for that day. Thankfully, an amazing, consistent substitute was able to cover for me for an hour and a half, so on my break, Aaron picked me up to take me to this appointment. Wanting to multitask, I told him to go grab lunch while I went through what I thought would be a quick procedure. After all, I had made it through the HSG in radiology with the medical personnel saying "wow" and gawking at my tumor. This would be no big thing. Right? Wrong!

Not long after I had hopped onto the table fitted with a cloth robe and put my legs in the stirrups, I got the familiar pain of the catheter. I had not quite realized how sore I was internally, but before I knew it, I was screaming out in pain. And no, I am not a demure or quiet screamer. Much like my facial expressions, my emotions are out there for all to see and hear. Think about this small fertility center, with a waiting room full of hopeful women looking for their miracle answer, and me yelling like Kate Capshaw in *Indiana Jones and the Temple of Doom.* As the male fertility specialist continued to probe the catheter deeper, he asked where it hurt, right or left? I screamed out at him, not so nicely, that it hurt everywhere. For what felt like hours, although it was minutes, the water shot up to finish the x-ray. When it was over, I was in too much pain. My husband was immediately rushed in, and when I felt like I could stand up, we went back to see the specialist with the x-ray. The tumor was huge, and it was in a place that could be causing severe side effects. It needed to be removed. I felt vindicated, as I had known there was something wrong with me. Having done the research, I listened as the specialist explained the types of procedures I could go through. I'll turn to the experts at WebMD to relay what I had so quickly tuned out in my mind:

> Myomectomy is the surgical removal of fibroids from the uterus. It allows the uterus to be left in place and, for some women, makes pregnancy more likely than before. Myomectomy is the preferred fibroid treatment for women who want to become pregnant. After myomectomy, your chances of pregnancy may be improved but are not guaranteed.
>
> Before myomectomy, shrinking fibroids with gonadotropin-releasing hormone analogue (GnRH-a) therapy may reduce blood loss from the surgery. GnRH-a therapy lowers the amount of estrogen your body makes. If you have bleeding from a fibroid, GnRH-a therapy can also improve anemia before surgery by stopping uterine bleeding for several months.
>
> Surgical methods for myomectomy include:
>
> Hysteroscopy, which involves inserting a lighted viewing instrument through the vagina and into the uterus. [Obviously, this one was out since I wanted to have a baby.]
>
> Laparoscopy, which uses a lighted viewing instrument and one or more small cuts (incisions) in the abdomen. [You know all those vaginal-mesh commercials you see that sometimes also include surgery from uterine fibroids? Just replaying those in my mind deterred me from this surgical method. Plus, my tumor was not small, and it was growing larger every day.]

Laparotomy, which uses a larger incision in the abdomen. [Bingo, this would be the one. But what did it entail?]

The information below, again from WebMD.com (http://www.webmd.com/women/uterine-fibroids/myomectomy-17717), helped me understand a little bit more about what to expect from this type of surgery.

Laparotomy is used to remove large fibroids, many fibroids, or fibroids that have grown deep into the uterine wall.

Need to correct urinary or bowel problems. To repair these problems without causing organ damage, laparotomy is usually needed.

What to Expect After Surgery
The length of time you may spend in the hospital varies.

* Laparotomy requires an average stay of 1 to 4 days.

Recovery time depends on the method used for the myomectomy:

* Laparotomy requires 4 to 6 weeks.

Why It Is Done
Myomectomy preserves the uterus while treating fibroids. It may be a reasonable treatment option if you have:

* Anemia that is not relieved by treatment with medicine.
* Pain or pressure that is not relieved by treatment with medicine.
* A fibroid that has changed the wall of the uterus. This can sometimes cause infertility or repeat miscarriages. Before an in vitro fertilization, myomectomy is often done to improve the chances of pregnancy.

How Well It Works
Myomectomy decreases pelvic pain and bleeding from fibroids.

Pregnancy

Myomectomy is the only fibroid treatment that may improve your chances of having a baby. It is known to help with a certain kind of fibroid called a sub mucosal fibroid. But it does not seem to improve pregnancy chances with any other kind of fibroid.

After myomectomy, a cesarean section may be needed for delivery. This depends in part on where and how big the myomectomy incision is.

Recurrence

Fibroids return after surgery in 10 to 50 out of 100 women, depending on the original fibroid problem. Fibroids that were larger and more numerous are most likely to recur. Talk to your doctor about whether your type of fibroid is likely to grow back.

Risks

Risks may include the following:

- Infection of the uterus, fallopian tubes, or ovaries (pelvic infection) may occur.
- Removal of fibroids in the uterine muscle (intramural fibroids) may cause scar tissue.
- In rare cases, scarring from the uterine incision may cause infertility.
- In rare cases, injuries to the bladder or bowel, such as a bowel obstruction, may occur.
- In rare cases, uterine scars may break open (rupture) in late pregnancy or during delivery.
- In rare cases, a hysterectomy may be required during a myomectomy. This may happen if removing the fibroid causes heavy bleeding that cannot be stopped without doing a hysterectomy.

It was just a matter of when the procedure could be done, so I made an appointment to speak to my doctor when she returned from her vacation.

CHAPTER 4

Navigating the Infertility Forest

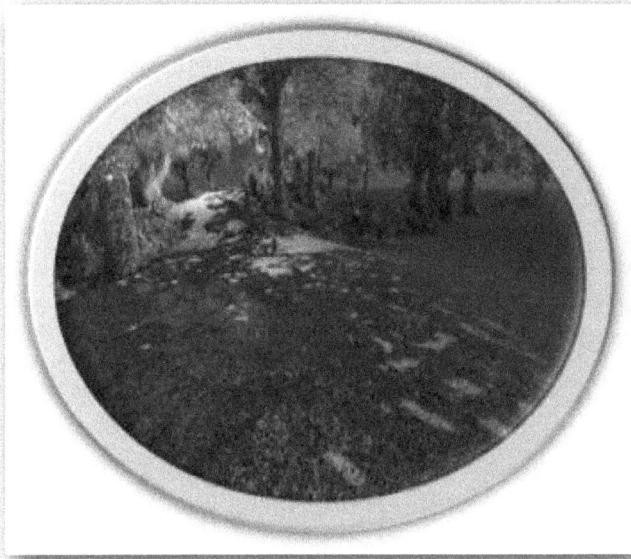

WE CONTINUED TO PROGRESS DEEPER down our road, desperate to get help from the all-powerful infertility wizards. I needed a clear uterus, and my husband needed some large veins removed from his testicles. A far cry from the brain, heart, and courage the characters needed in *The Wizard of Oz*, but here we were, trucking along farther down our own red-brick road.

Surgery. I had known it would come down to this. Hell, I had even advocated for it; however, the idea of surgery and the actual surgery deadline approaching were two different things. Not only was I dealing with the tentative date but I also had a new boss transitioning into my school. This was late July. As an administrator, I work twelve months. Although the summer is calmer, you never know what a new boss's expectations will be, so this was a lot of pressure on top of worry.

When I finally had my conference call with my specialist, she shared that she had talked to the hospital and it would either be early September or late October. Even though it would interfere with the start of the new school year, I hoped that the surgery would be earlier rather than later. Since I had been made aware of my tumor's foreign, abnormal, and growing presence, I had really started to develop more physical symptoms. If you like comedy and ever watched the movie *Spaceballs*, you have watched the scene where Bill Pullman and John Candy are in the diner when a customer heaves over in pain, only to have a space-alien-like creature erupt out of his stomach, growl, put on a top hat, and use a cane to sing "Hello My Baby" as he dances down the counter-top like Michigan Jay Frog. That is the type of thing I envisioned to be living inside me, except that, instead of my stomach, it was lodged in my uterus. It was the week back for teachers when the date of surgery was confirmed; it would be on September 3. The second-week students were in school. Once I knew that, little else occupied my mind.

A lot of people who are not in education have a misconception about what the job entails, especially over the summer preparing for the start of a new school year as an administrator. What it consists of is getting a building shiny, ready, and new for a hopeful, exciting school year. This entails a lot of filing, scheduling, planning, meeting, and answering questions. When teachers arrive the first week back prior to kids returning the following week, my priority becomes whatever their priorities are in order to get their classrooms ready, along with planning, implementing, and facilitating exciting and engaging professional development. It can be challenging to engage teachers in a separate location when all they want to do is get their classrooms set up and ready.

The reason I divulge all of this is that this was not an ideal time to be trying to prepare for a surgical procedure. With any hospital stay or surgical procedure, a lot of steps are needed before actually going "under the knife." This included a preoperation physical with my doctor, checking with my insurance to determine what would be covered, signing off on medical forms that basically stated that if I died it was not their fault, and donating blood to myself in case I needed it during the procedure. And because at this point my time frame was so short until the actual surgery, about three weeks out, I had to get all these things done ASAP.

If you ever watched the show *Seinfeld*, you know that Jerry Seinfeld did a brief comedy sketch during the opening of each show. In one instance, he talked about the waiting room at the doctor's office and how you go in and wait. Then, you feel excited when they call you back to the little room, but it is all about waiting in there as well. I've found that trying to call and actually speak to your doctor or the receptionist to schedule things is a similar, frustrating, and drawn-out process. This was especially true of my doctor's office, which had switched to an automated phone system that sent all calls to a prerecorded message. You see, at my doctor's office, they only have specific office hours, with an audio recording that comes on repeatedly to let you know that you are not calling within their scheduled time when you can actually speak to another human being. You can't even get the possibility of being connected to a live person until after 9:00 a.m. They turn off the phones during their lunch hour and a half, as well as at 3:30 p.m. And if the receptionist is busy—yup, you guessed it—right to the recording.

For me as an administrator, my office hours are from eight o'clock to four o'clock. I don't have a scheduled lunch or breaks, because these basically consist of whenever I have an opportunity to shove food down and take five minutes to go to the bathroom without being called on the walkie-talkie. For teachers, they have their students to think of and their classroom, which becomes their whole focus and world. Teaching is a profession that creates all other professions, so teachers have always been people I admire and hold in the highest regard. With that being said, for administrators, we have a whole school as our focus, which changes our perspective to a bigger, wider picture. However, we always have our "open door" policy. This means that if I'm your boss and you have an issue, question, concern, or just any kind of small talk that you want to do on the time you have allotted within your schedule, you can come in to interrupt what I'm doing, and I will push it to the side and focus on your priority. Think about a deli counter where you don't have to take a number. This made it extremely hard for me to get my doctor on the phone to schedule all my necessary procedures. I remember leaving three messages, and when I finally did speak to a human who hung up on me after I'd waited for twenty minutes, I was so frustrated that I left another message. I stated I was going to come in to schedule my appointment with my documentation that had the times I had called, the length of time I had to wait, and the names of the people I had spoken to. Shocker—after that message, I got a speedy call back, my forms filled out, and an appointment scheduled immediately. I hate to have to go to that "bitch" level, but unfortunately I always have that level inside me, and when someone is interfering with my health and well-being, it definitely comes out.

After all the steps needed before the procedures were set up, things moved very fast. With the pace of school and the growing tumor, I was on a constant merry-go-round of pain, worry, and anxiety.

It really hit me the day I went to donate blood. As things usually go in my life, taking blood was not an easy task. My veins are very difficult to find for some reason, and often when one is found, it doesn't like to give blood for as long as is needed. This always results in me being pricked on both arms and getting cotton-ball-taped souvenirs that everyone I pass throughout the day looks at with concern, asking what happened. And the passing out is always a fun side effect too. So unlike in my younger days when I tried to be a badass and stand directly after having my blood taken, I now sit there happy to drink the juice and eat the cookie. I have learned that drinking a lot of water helps, so on the day of my donation, I was well hydrated, nervous as hell, and of course had to hold my bladder.

Thankfully, I've learned to just be up-front about the challenges of my body when giving blood. I can always tell how seasoned a nurse is by his or her reaction: either sheer panic or "No problem, sweetheart." Luckily, that day I got the second one, which was good because I really had no idea what I was in store for. The nurse explained each step to me prior to doing it, which again I greatly appreciate. Logic helps me when I'm nervous and things are out of my control. This was not going to be the usual blood-taking process I had come to know. Instead, she had to get multiple units of my blood "just in case" something happened during the procedure and I needed a transfusion. I like to be prepared, but I didn't want to think about the possibility of something going wrong, so by then I was a bit of a mess inside. Thank God Aaron was there, but at that point, he was gripping my hand harder, so I knew his anxiety level was through the roof as well. There was also a TV in the background, and of course I was praying in my head, "Please, God, make my blood come out. Help me get this over with, because I do *not* want to go through this again." One unit of blood takes six to ten minutes. I swear it felt like days, but God answered my prayer, and it was successful. Again, I had mixed feelings: *Uh, woohoo to me having access to my own needed fluid if I start bleeding out on the table.* Like, how do you not worry after that, standard protocol or not?

The next few days leading up to the surgery were a whirlwind of worry and steps taken to get things in order—you know, in case I died on the table. I met with loved ones, got my life insurance set up so Aaron would be taken care of if something were to happen, did my best to get all work tasks done, and wrote some sappy, inspirational notes to send to people I loved prior to going into surgery. Whether it was psychosomatic or not, I really felt the pain of the tumor. It felt like it was protruding out of the bottom portion of my lower back and kidney area. I was in so much pain that I was vomiting and frequently had to lie down. Before I knew it, it was the night before the surgery. Since I had been in so much pain, I had to take a couple of days off work prior to the surgery. What to do the night before so as not to worry? Everyone said that the movie *Guardians of the Galaxy* was amazing, so we went and saw that. Then, we had some pizza out at a restaurant. Sadly, none of it made me forget the feeling of fear, dread, and anxiety that was now my permanent state. I had surgery in college on my knee, and the whole process was very rough. That and the liability paper outlining the possibility of death were plaguing my thoughts. When we got home, I went through my presurgical checklist. Nothing to eat or drink after ten. No big deal, right? I'd go to bed early; then I'd be getting ready for the hospital, so I wouldn't even have time to think of food, right? Um, wrong. I wasn't due to check in until noon the next day. It was torture not being able to eat, let alone drink anything. You never quite realize how much you need or enjoy having access to water until it is taken away. At four o'clock in the morning, I was absolutely miserable. Aaron, being the logical man that he can be in medical situations and wanting to solve my problem, told me to have an ice chip. He explained why the rule was in place to not eat or drink. It sounded good to me, so I gobbled up an ice chip, which quenched my thirst enough for me to fall asleep.

Of course I couldn't sleep in, so the next morning, I was up and ready to go. Next step on the checklist was to take off all jewelry. No problem. I took off all my rings—except, uh-oh, I guessed that included my belly-button ring. I had gotten this belly-button ring when I was twenty-six, as a reaction to a horrible breakup. I had not even attempted to take it out since then. It wouldn't budge. Aaron tried; it didn't even seem like it had the capability of coming off. To YouTube, where we watched an informative video on how to take out a belly-button ring. We tried this method, but it was no luck. Now, I was so anxious that they were not going to be able to do the surgical procedure because I couldn't get my belly-button ring out. But Aaron, always the voice of reason, told me that he was sure the nurse who would prep me for surgery had seen this multiple times and would be able to get it off. Anxiety relieved—for the moment.

Then, we were off to the hospital. I had my bag packed, had kissed my animals good-bye, and had my brightly painted fingernails and toenails to look at. It was only after I had gotten my bright-orange manicure and pedicure that I read the presurgical checklist, which said nail polish had to be removed. But I was too determined to keep a positive attitude, so I figured if they needed to remove it, they would. My mom and mother-in-law were both on their way to meet us at the hospital. I knew my mom would be freaking out, and lately, more than ever before, I found my mother-in-law's emotionless, logical, and medical approach to be quite comforting.

After checking in with the nice lady at the registration desk, I got my ID bracelet. If you've ever had surgery, you know just how many times you will be asked for your identification. Considering my last surgical procedure was on my knee and I was out of the hospital after the procedure, I had no idea what I was in for. I had to repeat my name and birth date every four hours while in the hospital. Oh, what fun!

Then, it was off to see the nurse, who quickly went through the steps of discarding my clothes and changing into the fashionable cap and gown. I explained the saga of my belly-button ring, and after I complied with the changing procedures, she removed the ring like the expert she was. I told her she could just throw it away. After all, what did a thirty-three-year-old need with a belly-button ring? I knew she had been doing this for quite a while as we made small talk. She was stern but kind and sensed my anxiety about the procedure, so she attempted to put my mind at ease. She also put my fingernail/toenail worry to rest when she said I could keep the nail polish on. Whew! I'd be able to have some semblance of sunshine as I went through this.

It wasn't long before Aaron was let back to sit with me, followed by my mom and his mom. You could sense the awkward nervousness from most of us collectively in the room. All my mom wanted to talk about and tell every medical employee that ventured into the room about was my "miracle birth" in the hospital and how I was premature. Having heard this story every year, specifically on my birth date and at the time of my birth (9:31 p.m.), I was certainly not in the mood on this day to hear it a million times, so I felt my anxiety clouded with annoyance. Thankfully, the anesthesiologist interrupted. My mother-in-law knew him from her days of working in the hospital, so that was a relief. After they caught up and made small talk, he walked me through the process of getting anesthesia. Good, because I definitely did not want to be awake at all for this. As Aaron squeezed my hand tighter and time ticked on, I knew he was feeling more and more anxious. Soon, two kind surgical technicians were at the door ready to escort me. I hugged and kissed everyone good-bye, expressing my love but holding my resolve to be strong. I of course was praying that it would not be the last time I saw everyone. Then, one last bathroom trip before I was escorted to the surgical room and asked to lie down on the cold metal table. Most of the surgical team was already in there with music blasting away. They had a good rapport going, and I liked the energy in the room. The anesthesiologist did his thing, and after I was asked a couple of questions, which I thought were small talk, I was out—I think even midsentence.

Chrissie's dreaded surgery, also known as a myomectomy, was finally upon us. We knew that the day was going to get to us. It was an impending event that we knew needed to happen, and yet we wished it was simply done and over with. Yet, through the natural progression of time, the date came. We were all understandably nervous, especially given the very complex nature of the procedure. It was not as if our doctor would be making a small incision in Chrissie's arm or leg. This was, for all intents and purposes, a C-section of a nonthinking organism. My wife's uterus was to be cut open, and a tumor the size of a large fetus was to be removed. We arrived at the Greater Baltimore Medical Center, where the operation was to take place. After the hospital staff got her in her cap and gown, we were made to wait until everything was ready for Chrissie's operation. My mom had shown up to counterbalance my mother-in-law's emotional reaction with her signature logic and reason. It was an event where I truly appreciated my mother's calm. Then Chrissie was taken back to the operating room.

That's fine, I thought to myself. *This is all fine. She is going to be fine.* I found myself thinking the word *fine* a lot, but that was—fine. I was told the surgery would take a couple of hours and that Chrissie would need some recovery time once the procedure was over. I understood all these necessary steps, and I thought I could handle the wait time. I thought I could handle it, that is, until about an hour and a half in. My mother and my mother-in-law were sitting at a table with me, making sparse conversation, and all the while I was overheating with anxiety. I literally felt like my brain was melting. Finally, the doctor came out and told me just how swimmingly the procedure had progressed.

"Your wife's uterus looks beautiful, and she is in the recovery area while the drugs wear off."

I thought I was going to fall over and punch the ground as I went down. "When can I see her?" I asked, in a voice that provoked a look from my mom.

"She still needs some time. I will come and get you when she is ready." The doctor exited stage left, and I stormed outside. I wanted to see my wife and make sure she was OK. Of course, that was not an option. I remember pacing around the outside of the hospital building and looking at the gardens and water features. I looked down at a tiny, well-kept pond that was right in front of the entryway to the building, and there were little koi fish swimming through it. I looked at those fish, feeling a sense of peace at first. Then, I got real pissed at those little guys. "You little assholes, swimming around in your damn pond. Just flitting to and fro, no idea what's happening in the building right next to you." Just as I was about to start punching the water like a moron, a nurse came out to see me.

"Your wife is ready for visitors!" she said jovially. I thought I was going to pass out. Instead, I dragged myself away from the koi pond and into the building to make sure my wife was OK. Those fish would live to see another day.

———❦———

Being under anesthesia is quite interesting. It is nothing that you can prepare for or even imagine. The tendency is to think you will be on a trip, one that is similar to being high. Having done drugs during my troubled youth, this was my misconception. Even though I had surgery in my college years, I didn't remember the actual experience of going under. I only remembered waking up disoriented and feeling like I was in a dark room surrounded by the presence of my friend who had passed away. Some people have explained it as being in a time machine: one minute you're there in a certain time; then you're gone, only to awaken in a whole different location and period. I read that another person compared it to being the closest to death that you can get. The latter two definitions are closer to what it is actually like. All I knew was that one minute I was nervous, talking to hospital staff and lying on the cold metal table. And the next minute, it was blackness. It felt like no time had passed for me when I awoke groggily in the hospital postanesthesia-care unit where I was being monitored by nurses. I remember waking up to see my doctor, who told me the procedure was a success. I felt like I was making perfect sense as I conversed with her, but I later found out that it was just gibberish and babble. Aaron came back soon afterward and sat with me as I dozed in and out of consciousness. Although I was numb and in pain, I felt like I had been given a new chance at life. I was so happy I had made it through the surgery that it was hard to feel anything other than renewed positivity.

It took hours in the postanesthesia-care unit before I was able to be transitioned to my hospital room. When I was finally able to transition, I was wheeled down so many different hallways and passages of the hospital that I felt like I was on a roller coaster, except I couldn't see what was coming in front of me because I was so strapped down. I had no idea there were so many secret passages and back doors for employees only within the hospital.

The most defining moment came when we got to my room. The orderly who had wheeled me was preparing to transition me from my metal slab of a cart to my hospital bed when I beat him to it and slid myself over. He was highly impressed that I had the strength to maneuver myself straight from surgery. Of course, Aaron was telling me to be careful, but for me it was like, "Oh, hey, there's my fighting spirit back." Then, it all came flooding back to me how I had overcome my knee surgery, recovering for six weeks in a dorm room during winter in Pittsburgh, the hilliest city there is. I felt strong again and was happy to be healthy. And the drugs weren't too bad either. Aaron slept that night in a very uncomfortable chair in my hospital room and continued to do so throughout my stay. If I didn't know how much he loved me before, it was truly evident during this time.

During my first night, I had the most amazing nurse, Betty. She was kind, caring, and also motivating. Every four hours, she would come in, check on my vitals, and ask me my pain levels, and a couple of times she even made me sit up and move my legs. At first when she asked me to sit up and move my legs, I thought she had to be kidding and said, "Seriously?" In response, she shared with me the importance of moving my legs, which included a whole bunch of medical side effects that I did not want to encounter. I also had to breathe into a clear jug for a set number of minutes, which I thought was odd but then took on as a personal challenge. The other fun part of my stay entailed the hospital putting a fluid collector in my toilet and keeping track of my urine. This became really annoying because every time I filled it up, I had to call to get it emptied. All that aside, I had made it through. I was alive, and the morphine certainly helped keep me in a euphoric state, numbing the pain and taking me off to a calm slumber.

The next morning, bright and early, the nurse awakened me and explained that she was changing out her shift. The other nurse came in, introduced herself, asked me to identify my personal information on my bracelet, asked me what procedure I had been there for, and took my blood. What a way to start the morning off. I felt the pain and was apprehensive about looking down. I didn't know what my stomach or scar would look like. The nurse explained the continued importance of tracking my urine. Lovely! She also shared that my bowels would take some time to regulate. This was an immediate concern for me. I remembered the constipation and pain I had experienced the last time I had gone through surgery, and that was just from my knee. I didn't have any idea how difficult it was going to be now, since my insides had been the target of the surgery.

She also shared that I could start eating. Woohoo! It seemed like forever since I had my last meal. Although the bowel issue made me apprehensive, it didn't stop me from checking out the menu. Pretty yummy-looking items for being in the hospital. I placed my order and visually checked out my room. I had a nice view out the window, access to my phone, and buttons on my hospital bed that turned the TV off and on. I was set. I wasn't looking forward to attempting to stand when I had to go to the bathroom, but I would cross that hurdle when I had to. Aaron had left early in the morning to go home to feed the cats. He seemed exhausted all around. It made sense, as I had watched him toss and turn in his uncomfortable hospital chair attempting to sleep most of the night. When my meal came, it tasted like the most delicious food ever. I know; hospital food—how could that be? It must have just been because I was so thrilled at the sight and taste of actual food. At that point it had been almost thirty-six hours since I'd eaten. Hell, the night before when I was told I could sip water, you would have thought it was the most expensive champagne with the excitement I felt as I saw it coming toward me.

I was able to have constant access to my phone, including social media. This was very nice, as I had been getting an outpouring of messages all expressing love, support, and prayers. It really made me feel grateful to have such wonderful people around me. When I had filled out what felt like a million forms prior to the surgery, I had been asked repeatedly about my religion and the name of my church. I realized why as I recovered. One visitor, a very kind elderly lady, brought me a blanket that had been made by my church to help me recover. Then, the new associate pastor, whom I had never met, came to my room to greet me and wish me well in my recovery. He was young, energetic, and very sweet. He seemed taken aback at my level of spirituality and faith. Not in a bad way, but just that I had such a positive attitude directly after getting out of surgery. I told him about the infertility struggle and also talked with him about the work I had done throughout my years at our church with the youth group, as well as facilitating the nondenominational service. Sometimes you just meet people you connect with on a spiritual level who are just cool and easy to talk to. This was one of those times. At that time, I had no idea the work he and I would do later on.

I had hungrily gobbled up my meal and drunk my juice and water. With all that I ordered, you would've thought I hadn't eaten in months. It was time, the moment of truth. I could no longer hold it and had to go to the bathroom. I shakily sat myself up. Whew, one part done. I then swung my legs over and stood on the floor. Thank God for the awesome hospital socks that kept my feet nice and cozy. Ouch, it hurt to stand up. With each small, slow step I took, I felt the pain of the scar, which reminded me of the current reality as to why I was in this room. Thankfully, the toilet seat was raised, and there were handle bars. When I was done, I felt like I had just accomplished a huge victory.

The next couple of days in the hospital, I fell into an easy routine and was the perfect patient. The medical staff shared that with me every chance they got, always as an excuse as to why they had not been more attentive to my needs, because they knew I was doing well. Aaron returned each night to stay with me. I could tell he was a wreck from worrying about my recovery. Little things like walking to the bathroom and washing up were extremely difficult. But I wore my pain like a badge. I had made it through the surgery and was ready to go home to embark on my six-week recovery. I felt positive about the future in front of me and blessed to be tumor free. I was disappointed though that I never actually got to see the tumor. I'm sure it was really gross looking, but after something lives and grows inside you, it's a morbid curiosity to see its makeup.

I only hoped that I would be back in the hospital soon delivering a baby in the same procedure instead of a tumor. As my doctor explained to me when she shared how much of a success my surgery was, they deliver the baby through a Cesarean when you've had this procedure in order to clear out the built-up scar tissue. She also shared that my ovaries and uterus were beautiful. *Um, that's great, I think.* I was elated when she told me that I was well enough to go home. I couldn't wait to be at home with my cats in my bed, watching some really awesome TV. It was a lingering worry that I had not yet had a bowel movement, but I pushed that to the back of my mind and chalked it up to it being difficult to go in the hospital. I was sure I would have more luck once I was in the comfort of my own home, right? The more I tried to convince myself, the more I knew it would be a problem.

Woohoo, checkout day! Once again, I started my day by having to give my name, my birth date, and a short summary of the procedure I had endured. The woman who did my checkout that morning, though, was powerfully unattractive and very unpleasant. She was sick and coughing uncontrollably. She made no attempt to respond to my pleasant small talk and instead stuck me quite violently in the vein to take blood. That was going to leave a bruise, I already knew. It must have been a sign to me that it was time to go.

After I got my final medication and dosage instructions, the orderly arrived to wheel me out. Apparently, they have to wheel everyone out after a surgical procedure and inpatient hospital stay, no matter what the patient's capability of walking is. I was elated when I saw the car. *Get me out of here!* As soon as I got home, I changed into comfy clothes and crawled into bed. The animals were a mixture of anxiety ridden and excited to see me. It was so weird though, because all the cats wanted to do was to crawl, walk, and curl up directly on my scar. It required constant redirection. There continued to be a stream of texts, calls, messages, and visits offering positive support. My mom was amazing and there every second she could be. Her friends were as well, and her best friend bought us the most fabulous Italian takeout dinner the first night I was home. It was the best thing I had tasted in a long time. I seemed to appreciate the little things more than I did before.

As I was taking my medication each day, I was still very concerned I hadn't had a bowel movement. When Italian food and prune juice made no impact, I went into freak-out mode. Aaron, being the calm problem solver, immediately ran out to the drugstore. They told him this medicine would make me go to the bathroom within the hour. Knowing my body's stubbornness, whenever anyone gave a specific timeline of what my body's reaction would be, it completely opposed that. I wanted to believe, but as the minutes ticked on and my discomfort level became raised in alignment with my worry, I went into full-on freak-out mode. Back to the drugstore went Aaron. This time he returned with Ex-Lax. Thank God the premiere of the season was coming on for *Sons of Anarchy*. At least I could focus on the dramatic twists and turns of the biker gang, along with Jax's sexy abs. Twenty minutes in, and I practically tripped over myself trying to get to the bathroom. It is amazing the bargaining you end up going through when you feel constipated. Without being too disgusting or graphic, it was a long bout in the bathroom filled with sweating, prayers, and crying, but no success. I wondered if my intestines would ever work well again. How on earth could there still be no bowel movement coming out with Italian food, prune juice, prescription drugs, and medicine? Again, I was thankful for the TV show. I lay as still as humanly possible, took my happy prescription pill that knocked me into dreamland, and fell asleep praying that the morning would bring some relief. The next day my prayers were answered. Whew! I did not have to call my doctor freaking out. Thank you, Lord!

My recovery went smoothly, and it wasn't long before it was time for my postoperation visit. After she told me how nicely everything was healing, I was shocked when my doctor launched into the IVF regimen she wanted to put me on right away. Wikipedia says the following about IVF:

> **In vitro fertilisation** (or **fertilization**; **IVF**) is a process by which an egg is fertilised by sperm outside the body: in vitro ("in glass"). The process involves monitoring and stimulating a woman's ovulatory process, removing an ovum or ova (egg or eggs) from the woman's ovaries and letting sperm fertilise them in a liquid in a laboratory. The

fertilised egg (zygote) is cultured for 2–6 days in a growth medium and is then implanted in the same or another woman's uterus, with the intention of establishing a successful pregnancy.

Whoa, my brain was having a hard time processing as my doctor continued to spout out details of the medication regimen. I'd had the surgery, and Aaron was scheduled to have his surgery so that we could have a natural baby. I didn't even know how I felt about IVF. I had an exasperated look on my face, and once I got my wits about me, I stopped my doctor midsentence. I explained that we wanted to try on our own, since I'd had the surgery and the complication that had been the tumor was removed. She paused and then said in a matter-of-fact tone: "It is highly unlikely that you will ever be able to conceive on your own."

What? Really? Seriously? No! I'm Christian. Miracles happen every day. Come on, God; prove them wrong. She went on to explain that miracles do happen that cannot always be explained, but in our case and scientifically again, it was highly unlikely we would ever conceive on our own. Even with Aaron's surgery? Yes, highly unlikely. I went on to talk about the possibility of us fostering to adopt. My doctor said that however we wanted to create our family, she supported us. But she also gave me the folder of IVF information just in case I changed my mind.

My mind circled around her words. I filled Aaron in on the conversation in the car. He too was flabbergasted. I guess we stubbornly believed that if we did all we could do, we would somehow be able to manage the easiest thing a man and woman are supposed to do when they have sex: make a baby. While he returned to work, I slipped into bed feeling defeated, frustrated, and above all *angry!* It was one thing for me to say for years when I was single and struggling to find Mr. Right that I was going to foster to adopt. It's not like I didn't mean that. I loved kids. Me, the advocate, teacher, and administrator. I would love to take in a child whom someone else deemed unlovable. But saying it and having it be one of my only options to be a parent were very different realities. I really wouldn't be able to have my own baby without medical help? I felt like such a failure as a woman. So I did the one thing I always do when I'm deflated: called my mom. She was equally upset and started to justify how it just could not be true. Feeling mildly comforted, I hung up the phone. There it was—the IVF folder, which consisted of this really adorable baby on the front smiling at me. Not today, baby, not today. I promptly took that folder and threw it across the room.

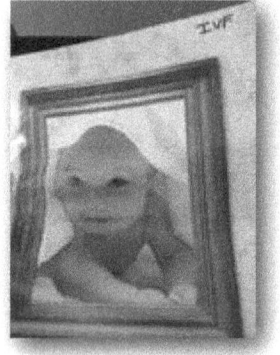

Then, I threw my head on the pillow and sobbed for what felt like hours. No words could do the feelings justice, but it felt like one of my dreams had just died.

My urologist, a pretty blond woman, was examining my testicles. She was doing it right there in front of my wife, and she had begun the process as though she were examining a cut on my finger. I felt my eyes flash all the way open as she pulled down the waistband of my boxers. I looked over at Chrissie, completely unsure as to how I was supposed to react to something like this. Chrissie, in unusual form, was doing her level best not to look at me. She was actually trying to pull off that thing you see in movies where the actor will be inexplicably staring at the ceiling while something highly uncomfortable is happening just feet away.

I remember thinking, *Chrissie! Chrissie, help me!* But alas, to no avail. The urologist's gloved hands began to make their way around my private area, and I was really unsure what to do here. I mean, this wasn't the first time that I had been examined. I was twenty-seven and had been through the military, so of course I'd had my balls examined. I had not, however, had them examined by a pretty doctor while my female partner was right there next to me. A part of my brain struck up some classic "bow-chicka-wow-wow" music, and I had to then very fervently fight the urge to get turgid. That may sound ridiculous, but until you are put in my shoes at that moment, I feel like any judgment needs to cease and desist. The urologist felt around and said, pretty much immediately, that I had a couple of serious varicocele. Which is to say that I had a couple of honking huge varicose veins in my scrotum. I pulled my pants up, and the doctor, pulling her gloves off, said, "Really, the only side effect of this condition is infertility." She was giving us a lopsided, sad smile. Trying to convey, I think anyway, that it was a tragic situation but not unmanageable.

"How do we, uh…you know…" I was being awkward as all hell for reasons already mentioned. "Ehem, fix this; how do we solve this problem?" I sputtered while waving my hand around my genitals.

Continuing with her smile that seemed to lean a little to the left, the urologist said the dreaded word that most people wouldn't want to hear in a doctor's office, "You are going to need surgery."

Of course I was. Because of course I was! That was just so exactly the path I had been blazing. One stupid goddamned complication after another. First, Chrissie had her surgery to remove a softball-sized tumor from her uterus, and then I needed surgery to remove tendon-sized veins from my nuts. Awesome! I did a face-palm action, which garnered some sympathy, but I didn't care. Why couldn't it just have been something easy? Why couldn't it be a pill I had to take for a month or two and then just be OK?

I had never had actual surgery before. I had never been anesthetized. My longest stay at the hospital was when I was six years old and my dad had accidentally infected me with meningitis. It was long and terrifying and left me with needles and holes all over my body. At least that's what I remember from that event. It took place over twenty years ago, and my addled brain can have a hard time remembering such things. My most vivid memory of that time was when I was walking from my hospital room to the play area for the youngest kids in the hospital. There were little toy dinosaurs and playhouses with mismatched dolls that all clearly belonged to different sets. I shook my head, trying to rid myself of this odd flashback to earlier, equally unpleasant times. I was going to have to have real, actual surgery. The thought was so foreign to me.

Chrissie's hand was suddenly on my shoulder, and I remember suddenly galvanizing myself in that moment. Telling myself that no matter what, I was going to do this. I was going to do this for my wife and for my future kids. I was going to do this for my family, and there was no amount of fear that was going to sway me from that path. I remember driving home from the doctor's office and feeling an odd, surreal sensation.

"Do I even have the right to feel like this?" I asked myself. "Should I be ashamed of myself for being so trepid about going under the knife?" I decided that I would not be scared. I would not be some mewling child afraid of what he did not know. I was going to go through all of this, and I was going to be fine.

Between the first doctor's appointment and the actual surgery date, there was a lot going on. I had my job as an additional assistant at Perry Hall Middle. It was a difficult but rewarding job, assisting differently abled kids through their daily schedule. I would act as a scribe, writing for the kids who needed it as they told me what they wanted on their worksheets and tests, and what have you. I would also reread instructions and maintain the focus of the students, as they tended to list off into their own minds. But then, Chrissie had found me a job at a Title One school in Randallstown as a paraeducator. This was a job that would pay twice as much and really utilize my skills as an educator. I would work across multiple grade levels and be instrumental in testing students' reading abilities.

But of course, the surgery was looming. It was hanging over my head like a dark rain cloud in those stupid antidepressant-medication commercials. It was funny, because the school that had hired me to be a paraeducator needed me to sign my contract. They needed me to do that the day of my surgery. I felt so dumb, walking into the school where I would be working in sweatpants and a hoodie. I apologized more times than I could count to the secretary and then also to the assistant principal. Everyone assured me that it was OK and that there was no offense taken, and I'm sure they meant it, but I still felt like an ass. I sat down and looked over the contract as quickly as possible, only wanting to get back in the car with Chrissie, who was idling outside. I signed every line and initialed every dash, just trying to do everything as quickly as possible. The neck of my hoodie started to feel really hot as I sat there looking over all the details. The surgery was drawing ever closer, minute by minute, and sitting there in that damned hot office that was essentially to be my future place of work felt sweltering.

I signed the last page and thanked the twelve-month secretary for her patience and acceptance of my less-than-OK appearance. She told me for probably the fifteenth time that it was OK, and I was fine and not to worry about anything. As quickly as possible, I got my sweaty self out of that building and into the car. Chrissie was all smiles when I got in.

"How did it go, honey?" she asked. Her gorgeous smile reached each ear in a way that really allowed me to forget the embarrassment that was my interaction with the secretary and the upcoming horror that was my surgery.

"It went!" I said, scratching around my collar and pulling at the waistband of my sweatpants.

"Good!" Chrissie said, putting the car into drive and heading for the first surgery of my life. The facility was not very far away, and we found the specific building where my surgery was to be held rather easily. We pulled into the parking lot and got out of the car. My mother and youngest sister, Alli, arrived a few minutes later in support of my and my wife's mental health. They were relatively successful. The first part of the procedure was to have some blood drawn in the event that there was a complication during the surgery. That, I found, was extremely worrying, and I suddenly felt like an ass for being so nonchalant about the moments leading up to Chrissie's surgery. The blood was being drawn, and I, being the moron that I am, looked over at the syringe as it was being filled with the precious liquid that allowed my body to move and breathe and, you know, generally exist. That's when the sickness hit me. A wave of nausea more powerful than I had felt in quite some time.

The nurse who was drawing blood apparently noticed my face blanch and asked for some assistance from other employees there. I vaguely remember Chrissie's eyes widening as she saw the blood drain from my face and another nurse fanned me with a nearby notebook.

Both nurses were obviously veterans of their craft, because they conversed among themselves that they had done this very same thing three times already today. And each time they had administered said treatment, it was to a young, strapping gentleman such as me.

Ha! I remember thinking while I was sitting in that reclining chair. *You can't make me feel stupid!* A gout of bile threatened to make its way up my throat; I fought it down with difficulty. *I already feel stupid! I feel stupid because I am actually pretty dumb! So there!*

One nurse continued to draw my blood, and the other continued to cool me off with her improvised fanning device. When the initial procedure was all done, I was led to a room where I was handed the classic paper hospital gown and cap. I'm sure most if not everyone reading is at least a little familiar with said object. It's obscurely difficult to put on: your ass is hanging out for everyone to see, and if you are a guy with a big dick (not bragging, just saying that it's not small), you have a lot of—I don't know—man cleavage hanging out there. So there I was with the dumb cap and gown standing in the middle of the facility. My butt was feeling the cool breeze of the air conditioning, and my penis was swinging to and fro underneath my damn gown. I stood there for quite a few minutes actually. Not because of any hesitation of my own, but because my doctor (the pretty urologist from earlier), my anesthesiologist, and my nurses just weren't ready. I stood there awkwardly, a twenty-seven-year-old man with his hairy butt nigh on hanging out of this stupid paper gown. Finally, a male doctor whom I had not yet seen walked up to me, dressed as one would imagine a doctor to be dressed. He had scrubs on with latex gloves covering his hands and a cap that was of the same make and model as my own. He grabbed the flaps of my gown and pinned them together with the swiftness of a very practiced hand.

"There you go, buddy," he said, a wry smile on his face. "If everyone is going to get a show, they should pay for it, right?"

I blushed more deeply than I thought possible and mumbled, "Yeah, my wife wouldn't be too happy either." The doctor gave a jovial Santa Claus laugh and jaunted on over to one of the counters to fill out doctor stuff on a clipboard.

After it was clear that I wasn't going to be seen for a moment or two, the office staff sat me back down in the chair where my blood had been drawn. Chrissie was there again, and I was starting to feel the sensation of near motion sickness again. Finally, my urologist popped her head into my waiting area. She looked really tired and bereft of rest or even spirit, really. She had bags under her eyes, and her face was, I think, more pale than mine. She gave me a quick explanation of how the procedure would go, and Chrissie was there listening to everything right next to me, her hand on my shoulder. I remember my urologist saying something about the surgery involving a microscope, which I found a little worrisome. Despite that, I kept cool externally. Or at least I like to think that I did. I don't know; my mind was everywhere, and suddenly there were needles in my arms again.

I was being told there was nothing to worry about and that I would be OK. I remember being wheeled into the operating room and being told that there was nothing to worry about. It was odd; the drugs were starting to kick in, and I could feel a wave of heat wash over my pelvis and then my chest and then—nothing. Literally nothing. I try to recall even one small detail. Maybe a dream, maybe a moment of consciousness during the actual surgery. (Well, thank God that didn't happen, I guess—right? Ha! Ugh.) But no. There was nothing. I was looking at the face of one of the nurses, and next I was waking up to my wife sitting next to my hospital gurney. I was still garbed in the paper gown and cap. The disorientation was unreal. My head was spinning as though I had been on a twelve-hour bender. Apparently I had said something to the effect of "Oh no, it's not even second period yet. Where is Stewart?" Before coming to and having my pupils surge back into focus, I had also reacted quite poorly to the aftereffects of being under. I found myself lumbering around like a little white Bigfoot. But at the end of the day, I got home and in bed. I remember, just as I was falling asleep, looking down at my surgical site and thinking to myself, "Ow! I look like an angry elephant down there." Then sleep.

CHAPTER 5

The Emerald City of Fostering to Adopt

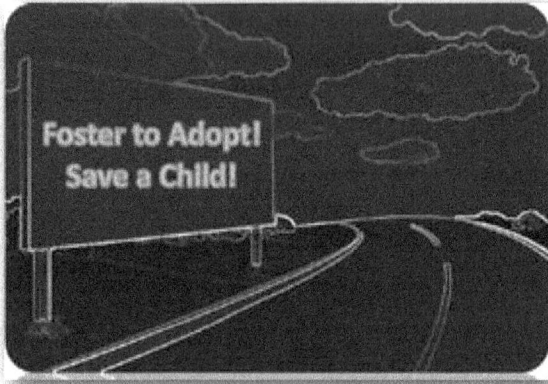

Months passed after Aaron's surgery in November. Still no luck with conception. Each month, I prayed that Aaron's motility had gone up. But sperm are very interesting—not in the ways you would imagine or joke about. They are a lot trickier than I ever realized. Not only are they impacted by certain characteristics of your lifestyle but, even if you make changes to your diet, sleep schedule, or exercise regimen, or in this case have a varicocele repair done, it also takes any changes at least three months to show up. This waiting all the while getting my period every month was becoming ridiculous. As time continued to march on, Aaron had his motility tested at least four times within the appropriate three-to-six-month time frame after surgery. The motility went up by 2 percent. But after the moment we had to celebrate the slight increase, at his next test it went back down, leveling at a pretty consistent low motility rate. I never thought I would care so much about sperm count and motility percentages in my life. I continued to pray that we would somehow get a miracle and one month I just wouldn't get my period; however, it never came to fruition. Each month another red-brick road along with my hopes faded away. Eventually, I started to feel numb to it. No more taking action, just complacent with life as it was.

Having our own baby seemed like an unrealistic possibility, so we started discussing adoption. Where did we even start? I looked up fostering to adopt and the state agency along with coincided information. Friends who had adopted out of the country shared information and resources with me. For us, it just seemed unnecessary to go out of the country with all the statistics when several students I encountered were in foster care. After all, I saw those articles and commercials about making your home a permanent one for a child in a temporary situation. We could do that! Aaron and I just wanted to be parents. We didn't care if the child was our blood. Even though this was the consensus we were coming to, we still had no idea where to begin and were so depleted from the lack of success. We felt like we had already given so much with so little success. Day by day time passed, along with our motivation to take action.

As fate would have it though, I had been dealing with a "spicy" child at my school. That's my name for students who have what other people perceive to be "behaviors." My philosophy is that kids exhibiting "spicy" behaviors are only asking for love in the unloveliest of ways because they don't have the tools to advocate for themselves with their emotions. This is where I come in. For whatever reason, God has gifted me with the ability to get through to kids in tantrums, crises, and so on. Well, I had one who was truly challenging me. She was a cute, blond first grader who had already been transitioned to three different teachers because she could not keep her hands to herself and wanted to do whatever she wanted to do, which of course was not her actual school-work. Throughout the year, she and I had seriously bonded. She was teaching me just how far my patience level could stretch as she introduced me to what it was like to truly interact with a child with oppositional defiance disorder.

I basically became the only person in the school who could get her to deescalate. She had a strange fascination for a bizarre video game that she played all night. This was all that she would want to talk to me about, along with some other more concerning information, about which I had to consult with outside resources on how to appropriately handle.

One day, I was in the midst of facilitating an IEP (individualized education program) team meeting when my principal came to the door, a distraught look on her face, needing me to step out. When I did, she shared with me what had happened. My girl had gone into the boys' bathroom, gone into a little boy's stall with him, and proceeded to take off all her clothes except for her underwear in order to do "sex things." It was a very hard situation all around, as we had to investigate both students. The little boy was in foster care. After going through the appropriate steps of the investigation, we consulted his foster parent along with his caseworker and therapist, who came to visit with him at the school. I had a positive rapport with his foster parent, who had been a longtime parent of the school. As we ended the conference and made pleasantries with small talk, it occurred to me that I should ask her how she ended up working with foster care. So me being me, with heartfelt bluntness, I changed the topic of conversation to one that was more personal and asked her what the process was like, explaining that my husband and I wanted to foster to adopt. She was moved and immediately started sharing the steps with excitement. She told me all about the private agency that she worked with and enthusiastically recommended I give them a call.

What was this feeling in the pit of my stomach? It had been so long since I felt it. Hope—excitement at the potential of something good happening. Oh, how I had missed these feelings. I had previously called the state department to inquire about the process of fostering to adopt, but I had not heard back from them. When I called this agency, however, I immediately got a pleasant, excited, kind young woman on the phone. She shared all the information about the program and the process. By the end of our call, I had the orientation meeting set up for Aaron and me. This just seemed like the right track. After all, what were the odds that a situation at my school was going to lead to this? It had to mean it was meant to be. At least that is what I told myself as we embarked on the journey over the next several months of jubilantly skipping down the red bricks of our road, passing each speed bump in the process with flying colors. It truly seemed like fostering to adopt would be the way, and the elusive Emerald City that we had been so determined to get to was at the end of our infertility road.

After the orientation meeting, we received a foster-parent handbook, along with a mound of paperwork and an outlined training schedule. This was definitely going to keep us busy throughout the entire summer, as it entailed attending twenty-nine hours of required training from six to nine every Tuesday and Thursday, along with a first-aid and CPR class. It didn't matter. We were ready to do whatever it took.

I was anxious and apprehensive for the first class. I had to attend by myself, as Aaron was finishing up a college course. I was greeted kindly by the young woman who had done the orientation. She continued to convey charisma and a sincere, caring demeanor. I was pleasantly surprised that they had dinner available with drinks, sides, and dessert. How nice! I sat next to the only other person who had been in our orientation. She and I made small talk and sat, both anxiously unsure of the information that was about to be presented to us. The presenters introduced themselves and their roles. Then, there were some icebreakers where we all learned more about one another. After this activity and the discussion started to get rolling, I felt at ease. With schooling in my life, I hadn't really found my niche until graduate school, with the topics of most of my courses being teaching, leadership, and administration. I thrived within those courses and throughout those topics. Within this training, I was finding the same level of enthusiasm. ADD (attention deficit disorder) is a funny thing, especially as I've gotten older and have learned strategies to manage it so I can be professional. When there is something that I have no interest in, time passes very slowly, and I have to keep myself engaged through taking notes. But with topics of interest and passion, as this training was turning out to be for me, I felt engaged and invigorated by the discussion, and the time went very fast. When I got home, the people and discussion were all I could talk about, excitedly recounting every minute to Aaron.

On the third training class, he finally got to come with me. By that point, it felt like all the participants were family, because through our discussions, we had shared so much of our personal lives. I will say that I had never encountered such kind people in my life. They were each so considerate, loving, real, and open about their experiences. Whether they worked in the health-care industry or drove a van to pick up people with disabilities, I felt like my life was enriched just by meeting them.

After Aaron came for the first time, he seemed to feel the same sense of purpose and excitement that I did. We could come home each time from a long day of work and be riveted by the trainings, chatting until all hours of the night about the content. For the first time in a long time, we were acting like two giddy teenagers. The twenty-nine hours of training that we navigated that summer included the following topics:

* Handbook Review: We reviewed all agency expectations and COMAR (Code of Maryland Regulations) during this class. We also reviewed the process of them placing a foster child, agency expectations in regard to working with biological families, and terminating biological parental rights with a foster child.
* Placement: During this class we reviewed placement procedures and referral trends. During this training participants were introduced to what an FTDM is. The purpose of FTDMs prior to placement and during placement was covered. An additional review of foster-parent responsibilities including participation in visitation with family was also focused on.
* Reasonable and Prudent Parenting: This class reviewed the reasonable and prudent parenting strategies. During this class family visitation was discussed. The benefits of family involvement are reviewed and the foster parents are given multiple case scenarios during the class.
* Professional Communication: Since we as foster parents would be working with multiple team members including medical professionals, therapists, family members, DSS (Department of Social Services) workers, agency workers, lawyers, and school staff, professional communication was addressed during this class. This class covered how to communicate in a professional manner even when concerns arise.

- Human Development: This class covered the stages of human development and sexual development as well as typical versus atypical development. They also reviewed disabilities such as autism, Down syndrome, fragile X, fetal alcohol syndrome, and intellectual disabilities.
- IEP: Since this agency was "therapeutic foster care" many of the kids had IEPs, so they did a brief overview of the IEP process, parent surrogacy, along with how to advocate effectively. During this class foster parents were informed about the importance of including biological families in these meetings.
- Trauma: This class covered the impact of trauma on the children placed. It addressed behaviors that parents may encounter and reviewed trauma-informed strategies.
- Self-Awareness: This class focused on how foster parents' own personal beliefs, values, motives, and desires could impact their parenting. They discussed fears of doing foster care and misconceptions about biological families. In addition, ways to incorporate children's beliefs, customs, and values into the foster family even when differences arise. Foster parents completed the True Colors Personality test. They also discussed the results of the test and how some of their traits may be an asset or something they need to be mindful of when working with others.
- Managing Disruptive Behavior: This class provided foster parents with an overview of the difference between discipline and punishment. They stressed that every behavior has meaning and that, in order to successfully address behaviors, the child must feel safe and secure and trust the foster family. Strategies to build this trust were also reviewed. Finally, they discussed how to deal with kids running away, as well during appointments, since this is when an increase of incidents of negative behavior occur.
- Children's Mental Health: During this class foster parents were introduced to children's mental health. They discussed common childhood diagnoses, suicide, and crisis planning.
- Working with Biological Families: During this class the benefits of family involvement, the legal process of foster care, permanency

planning, what to expect following visits, expectations of foster families, and strategies for foster parents to use to ensure biological families are kept involved and informed were shared.

* Human Trafficking: This class introduced foster families to human trafficking, the warning signs, and preventive strategies.
* Safety: This class provided foster parents with home-safety information as well as car-seat information.
* CPR and First Aid.

The CPR course fell right on our anniversary, so we made a quick trip to Florida and returned to spend the night getting trained on how to properly administer CPR. We got a card and everything. Even though it wasn't what we envisioned for our three-year anniversary, we were definitely excited at the prospect that, on the following year, we might finally be parents.

Throughout the training schedule, we had been getting the necessary paperwork completed. Tackling the mounting paperwork and requirements needed to even be applicable to be a foster parent mimicked the process of buying a house. It included, for both Aaron and me, a DMV driving record (of course this cost a fee for each of us), an employer reference, five personal references, income verification, physical-exam documentation with a negative TB test, copies of our marriage license, car-insurance policy, homeowner's insurance policy, driver's license, most recent BGE bill, and mortgage statement. Along with providing all those copies, we also had completed our Child Protective Services background clearance, state and federal background clearances, and CPR and first-aid certification.

All those requirements are not what came to my mind when I thought about foster care and the stories I would hear surrounding it. But we were committed and had come through all of it stronger than ever as a couple, with a newfound excitement at the prospect of having children there to complete the empty parts of our hearts that were yearning for a family.

When you are given little lives to take care of for a short period of time, you are also given a very specific set of rules. This set of rules is rather extensive and, for the most part, rather hard to follow. One of the main rules given to people who have just started caring for children who are absolutely not their own is (obviously) "Seriously, don't hit them—that's not cool."

Chrissie and I found that to be a basic human right rather than a rule that needed to be described to us. I was confounded by the fact that our agency seemed to need to really emphasize that harmful physical contact was not OK. I figured that if you were going to go through so much training to become a foster or adoptive parent, it would be out of love; you wouldn't do it so you could be a neglectful sociopath. It struck me on many occasions that so many rules were in place for the purpose of not hurting the children they were trying to protect.

They outlined that, unless you're picking these kids up, giving them medical attention, or hugging them (which was actually kind of discouraged), you really aren't to put your hands on them at all. I was fine with all that stuff in the classroom and on paper. However, it was not as easy as it sounds, and I'll elaborate on why later.

The training itself was actually kind of fun. There would often be real-life conversation and discussion. Chrissie and I like to talk to people in settings like that, and it put us in a very good mood during and after training. I certainly did not see that coming. I was thinking it would be a classroom setting, and there would be desks in front of a projector board with a wheezy old lady at the front of the room sounding bored and like she was wondering why she wasn't retired yet.

It was in fact quite the opposite. I had missed the first night of training because of my college courses that I would later abandon entirely. Chrissie had simply gone without me. When she returned later in the evening, she was almost glowing.

"Wow, honey!" I remember saying. "I guess everything went well?"

Chrissie was all smiles and almost giggling as she recounted the events of her first evening at the private foster care agency. "It was amazing!" she declared, her cheeks flushed with excitement at the possibilities that our future held. "There were other people there who have already been foster parents and had so much to say! And the social workers did a really good job of just creating this dialogue about what it meant to be foster parents!"

I was ecstatic to see my wife so happy about this process that I had assumed would be an utter bore—an exercise in the mundane. I'm telling you, seriously, I did not want to do the stupid training.

Turned out my first night of training was actually kind of a blast. There was some food served that I found palatable; there was *Dr. Pepper* and chips and stuff. That was all fantastic! What really made the whole evening go well were the people who were training along with Chrissie and me. They were such a diverse group of people! Well, to be honest, they were all in their forties and fifties. Chrissie and I were the youngest there by a pretty wide margin. But there was a healthy mixture of white and black couples. I was absolutely the youngest one there though. It was weird. I mean, I was twenty-eight at the time. It was a little surreal at first, sitting in that room with all these people who had been through all this training and more. Hell, they were likely to do it all again. And there I was, a kid in his late twenties with his wife just trying to take care of some kids in need. I began to reflect on why I was there in that moment.

But then one of the social workers got up and began her introduction. Much to my surprise, she was a young one! Maybe in her early thirties! As I peered around the room, I realized that most of the social workers who were employed there were my age or just a little older. This was a weird thing to have focused on, but that is how my brain tends to work. I subconsciously try to find ways to ostracize myself. It is not the best way to function, but—that's my brain.

Once the social worker introduced herself to the room, she did the one thing that I hoped she wouldn't do. She noted that I was a new member to the group of trainees and asked that I say something about myself. Look, I'm not really a very shy person. I can be fun, open, and what have you. My issues begin with being the new guy. I hate that. It is the absolute worst! How do you navigate those situations without knowing your audience or pool of people you are forced to interact with? Well, there I was, in this ridiculous situation.

I was in the middle of a group of people who didn't know me and absolutely thought of me as a kid. And at the end of the day, I guess that's OK. But I really thought that, given the situation we were all occupying, maybe it would be best if these notions were left by the wayside.

I was in the marines. I had been through some pretty terrible shit. I had a lot of life experiences. It was almost as if I had started getting defensive before anyone had even asked me a question. I am an actual adult, not some "youth" just attempting a little life project. I found myself getting so angry before anything had really even gotten started. But then things actually got started. The other trainees didn't judge. They didn't act as though they were better than me. They didn't talk down to me. That was incredible! I suddenly thought that I was actually in a room full of people who did not judge me. And they truly didn't. It was an amazing feeling. They had all been through some terrible and incredible things. They had their own experiences. At the end of the day, they knew that I was there for a reason. They knew that I was there to help take care of a kid. That all Chrissie and I wanted to do was shepherd a tiny person to adulthood and have a happy and healthy life.

So we went from there. Each class had a different lesson. Each instructor had a different motivation for being there. We had one class that included a very in-depth idea about communication—the idea that just because you felt like you were making yourself clear, that didn't actually mean you were making yourself clear. We had another class that went in depth about why a child might react in a certain way to seemingly innocuous things. The lesson was very heavy on the idea that "Hey, you don't have any idea where this kid came from." So when they start losing their minds, just shut up and appreciate the fact that they might be processing something that you have never actually experienced before.

This was a lesson that I greatly appreciated. If only for the fact that I really believe in the idea that one does not ever really know what another person is going through. People are always in the midst of their own problems. Recently, I was working at a day camp in a town that was about twenty minutes away from me. I would show up on time for the most part, but given the situation my wife and I were in, that didn't always happen. On the mornings that I showed up late, there was a particular employee who would very sternly pull me over and say, "You are extremely late."

I would respond, "Yeah, I guess I am."

This employee would shake his head and say, "Go to the office and sign in as late."

This happened a couple of times too many. It especially became a problem on a morning when Chrissie had to endure a particular procedure. So when I showed up at 8:50 a.m. instead of 8:45 a.m., this fucking guy said, "You need to not get here so late. Go sign in as a late arrival." I finally lost it. I did not give a flying fuck about whether or not this asshole knew what was going on in my life. I let him have it.

"Oh, I need to not get here so late?" I asked. I was fucking livid. The guy seemed taken aback for some reason, as if the people who worked at this place didn't have lives or feelings outside of the camp. I watched as his stupid face became red and splotchy.

"Yeah, it's eight fifty," he said, as though I was some asshole kid who was just hungover and late because he didn't know what time it was.

"I was just at the fertility center." He got a quick look of someone who felt a little awkward. "I just got some news that wasn't all that great, and my wife and I are looking at a future without children."

This particular employee began to act rather uncomfortable. I furrowed my brow rather intensely to give a better idea as to how pissed off I was. "Look," he said, not making any eye contact with me at all, "I'm just saying that you are late."

That was not the best response for me. "And I'm just saying that you don't have any idea what I have been through today. I called my department head; she knows what's going on, and she is fine with it. You don't need to tell me I'm 'extremely late,' and you can just let me through and park and go to my job like a normal adult. So next time, maybe don't start off our morning with that type of interaction." Maybe that was a bit of a tangent, but it is absolutely something I believe in. You have no idea what people have been through, so don't interact with them as though you do, and don't start in with an exorbitant amount of hostility.

Anyway, I felt as though that was a very powerful lesson, and I was glad that we were being reminded of such a powerful message. I just wish that these people had been as knowledgeable in their actual practice as they were with their training. More on that later.

So yeah. The training had the habit of being awesome. We would talk about where we grew up and what it was like to be a kid in each individual environment. Chrissie talked about her life as a child of divorce. I talked about what it was like to have a parent become sick, then sicker, and then die. It was a very interesting situation, because it felt almost as if we were part of a support group. Other people spoke about their upbringings, and I was privileged to hear just how wildly different people's lives could be even if they were only a few miles away.

Training went on like that for a few months throughout the summer of 2015. Every session made me more hopeful for adoption and taking care of some kids who just needed a helping hand when no one else in their lives was willing or able to do so. When we finally completed training, it felt as though I was an actual adult! We all shook hands, and some of us even hugged. We had spent so much time together and shared so much personal information that it felt appropriate. We had really gotten to know one another. We loved the other members of our training pool, and we loved the social workers who had been there to impart their knowledge and experience. I truly wish that our perception had remained that way. It wasn't long before the positive feelings would give way to something much more in the opposite direction.

⁓

By now it was late August. We had started the process in June. We were ready for the next portion, which were the household requirements. This included a health and fire inspection of the home, participation in the SAFE home-study process, at least two home visits with our placement coordinator, and documentation of all pet vaccinations.

The SAFE study—wow, when I looked that up, it appeared to be that it was going to be a grueling emotional process for us to go through, having experienced trauma throughout different portions of our lives. The information from http://www.safehomestudy.org/SAFE/SAFE-Overview.aspx below outlines all that the process would entail.

SAFE is a structured home study methodology that allows child welfare agencies to effectively and systematically evaluate prospective families for foster and adoptive placement. Using research-based tools and processes, SAFE allows even the most novice Home Study Practitioner to do a thorough job evaluating prospective families.

There are Four Components to SAFE:

Information Gathering Tools

* SAFE provides practitioners with uniform information gathering tools that support the home study interview. These tools include **Questionnaire I, Questionnaire II,** and the **SAFE Reference Letter**. These tools aid the Home Study Practitioner in doing more targeted interviewing. The Questionnaires and Reference Letter assist the Home Study Practitioner in identifying strengths, as well as issues to be addressed early in the home study process, thereby eliminating a great deal of time "guessing and/or fishing" for issues that should be addressed or explored further.

Structured Analysis

* SAFE has identified 70 Psychosocial Factors that research has demonstrated to be necessary for safe and effective parenting - either through adoption, kin or foster care. The **SAFE Desk Guide** and **Psychosocial Inventory** provide an inter-related, supported and

structured process to assist Home Study Practitioners in determining the strengths and limitations of a particular Applicant Family.

PRE-FORMATTED HOME STUDY REPORT

+ The Pre-Formatted Home Study Report is uniform in its organization and appearance, but is tailored to each state or province's requirements. Each SAFE Home Study looks exactly alike while still meeting the needs of individual regulations, laws, and rules of a state or a province. Because of the uniform nature of the Pre-Formatted Home Study Report, the SAFE home study reader knows exactly where to look for the issues and strengths of the Applicant Family and how those strengths and/or issues might affect either a specific child or child yet to be identified.

THE COMPATIBILITY INVENTORY

+ The SAFE Compatibility Inventory helps support placement workers in determining the appropriateness of fit of an Applicant Family and the child or children in question.

SAFE is a structured evaluation process that assists practitioners in identifying and addressing both strengths and areas of concern that may impede current functioning as well as safe and effective parenting. SAFE provides Home Study Practitioners with a structured methodology that supports the social work interview as well as provides a uniform methodology of interpreting and assessing the information gathered during the home study process.

Of course, my first priority was to get to cleaning and ordering. They provided us with a list of things needed in order to pass the home study, such as a fridge thermometer, smoke alarms on every level of the house, a first-aid kit, nonslip mats in all the bathtubs, and a fire extinguisher. In addition, we had to have our emergency and evacuation plans prepared and in an area accessible to all who lived in the house. Being the sequence-oriented person I am, I diligently ensured we had completed each step. I was feeling purposeful, like all this work we had put in was finally going to lead to something.

And although the SAFE study interviews were emotionally grueling— Aaron and I were interviewed first together and for the remaining sessions separately—we at least felt like we had a good rapport with our placement coordinator who was conducting the survey. On our second visit, she brought up the possibility of us getting two girls aged four and ten. You can say that you love all kids, genders, and races equally. But you never really know how you feel until you are presented with becoming the parent of one. As strange as it may seem, as I am the palest, whitest woman in the world, I had always imagined that I would raise a black boy. To those who know me personally and have seen me interact with kids, this makes complete sense. So when I was presented with the chance to have girls, two of them, who were white, I was a little taken aback. I politely listened to all the details of their case, contemplating what it would be like to have two girls with such a wide age span. One of the girls had even been at Aaron's school where he worked in the prior year. After our coordinator left, I immediately looked the girls up. As I studied their faces, I imagined what it would be like to have them in our care: their likes, their dislikes, the activities we would do, and just the overall idea of getting to be their mom. The more the idea rotated around with the pictures of their faces fresh in my mind, the more I felt like it was the right move.

When we met with our coordinator again, we conveyed our enthusiastic interest. She explained the process with the courts: the girls had been in the foster-care system for three years, and their case was coming up on potentially terminating parental rights at a court hearing scheduled for October. Yes, this was what we as a pre-adoptive resource had wanted! She said she would reach out to their attorney and express our interest. Our SAFE study had concluded, and shortly after it went to the head of the agency, we got our official letter saying we were licensed foster parents. The images of the girls continued to play in my mind as I wondered how they were doing, how school was going for them, and when we would hear an update on their case. After hearing nothing for several weeks, we reached out to our coordinator, who shared that their case had been postponed until January because their father was fighting the termination of rights even though he had no means to take care of them. We were crestfallen. After we had processed the initial shock of potentially getting two girls, we had been very excited at the idea. Now what could we do? Wait, and be offered other potential cases in the interim to see if any of those would be a more appropriate fit. Great. Just what we wanted after this extensive process, more waiting.

Within the next month, we were presented with two cases. One was a five-year-old black boy with autism whose mother had been killed in a hit-and-run. This seemed like a good potential case, but our hearts just didn't respond with the same fervor as to the case of the two girls. The other was a seven-year-old white boy who had ADHD and ODD. This case ended up being for reunification, so we said no right away. We did not want to have to deal with the long, drawn-out process of having visits with the biological parent until rights were terminated. As hard as it was saying no to kids in need, we wanted to make sure we had the right situation for us, as we knew we couldn't handle giving the child up once he or she was in our care. It would be too devastating emotionally. So we continued to wait.

Remember the awesome new pastor who had come to visit me in the hospital? Well, he had met with me over the summer and convinced me to return to my church to help out with the high-school youth group. It had started in the fall, and I was definitely appreciative of the amazing high-school youth I got to meet, along with the distraction it provided. Each Sunday night, after watching football of course, I headed over to church for dinner, fellowship, fun activities, and devotions. Being in my church always provided me with a sense of love and peace. I continued to greatly need that feeling, as the fostering-to-adopt process was not moving in my timeline.

However, on Halloween, I really started to feel the impact of the emotional roller coaster of not having kids. I had gone to our teen Halloween party thinking it was going to be a fun event filled with everyone in costumes doing silly activities. And it was, but all the adults brought their adorable young children dressed up, and they were running around and enjoying the festivities. When we had been presented with the possibility that we could get two girls at the beginning of the month, I had stupidly imagined what it would be like seeing them get dressed up in their costumes and taking them trick-or-treating. The fact that our fostering endeavor was at a complete standstill combined with seeing all the adorable children running around the church where I had for so many years wanted to have a family of my own was too much. I felt the tears forming in my eyes and the sick feeling in the pit of my stomach. I made up a lame excuse and literally ran out of the church with my cat tail between my legs. The minute I got to my car, I called Aaron and my mom. The tears were flowing when I talked to Aaron, but when my mom got on the phone, they had progressed to full sobbing. There is just something about talking to your mom that makes the emotions really come out. Through my hysterical crying, I shared how hard it was, how every time I felt close to being a parent, it got ripped away from me. Of course, the faith-filled Christian that I am was at that point questioning why God was taking so long and what the purpose was for all this. I just felt so yucky! I wanted to curl up in bed and just sleep it all away.

Two days later as I was driving home from work, I got a call from one of the caseworkers within our agency. She shared that there was a five-year-old black girl with autism who needed a permanent home, as her parent had already signed rights over. I wondered if this was God. I had just been so upset, and here was a new possibility. After she shared more details, she told me to talk it over with Aaron to see if we wanted to have a meet and greet. I also of course looked her up as well. When Aaron heard her case and saw the picture, he was excited. We both felt like we should go ahead with the meet and greet, but even though we were trying to convince ourselves this was the right fit, in our hearts something was missing. For some reason, we just couldn't get those two other girls who had been presented to us initially out of our minds. Even so, we set up the greeting. The caseworker determined that the potluck Thanksgiving party would be the perfect opportunity. She said that she would arrange it so we could sit with the little girl. We convinced ourselves that this was it, and as the days passed closer to the meeting date, we became more nervous.

What do you wear to meet your potential future daughter? I wanted to make an impression without being too flashy or inappropriate, so I decided on my new blue-and-black-striped sweater dress. The event was located at the alternate location for the agency, which was further away than we were used to driving. The sky looked bleak and gray, and there was a massive swarm of black crows perched in the trees as we went to turn into the agency. I couldn't help but think it was a bad sign. We pulled into the parking spot alongside one of the other caseworkers whom we had come to know through training. She was one of our favorite people to interact with. After we greeted one another with small talk and pleasantries, she shared that, along with the girl we were meeting, the two girls we had initially been presented with would also be at the event. I felt my heart skip a beat. We would finally get to meet the two girls who had tugged at our heartstrings since we were presented with their case. But wait; we were here to meet another little girl, one who was more available. My mind knew that, but my heart kept focusing on the other two.

At all the trainings, the paperwork, food, and all other details had always been well managed. We were not early for this event, so it was quite surprising to see the employees scrambling around to organize the casseroles. There were no set seating arrangements, and the caseworker we were there to meet had not seemed to have any seating arrangement prepared. Nor could we find her with all the hustle and bustle. We politely asked someone if we could sit anywhere, to which the person replied that we could. As we scanned the room, lo and behold, there were the two human beings who modeled the pictures we had looked up for so long. I whispered to Aaron that I thought that was them. He agreed. After we got some punch, we decided to go over and sit with them alongside their foster mom.

It was surreal sitting near the two little faces we had only seen in pictures and imagined for over a month and a half. After a polite greeting, we made our introductions, only to realize that it was not just the foster mom of the two girls we were sitting with. It was their biological father and grandmother as well. And it turned out the girls' brother, who was placed with a different foster-care agency, was also in the room. He came over to sit with us as we ate. The foster mom's adopted daughter was also in attendance at our table. She was an eighth grader who had an outgoing personality, was stylish, and clearly did not want to be there. I enjoyed sitting next to her and bantering back and forth about school. We were all getting along so well that we hardly noticed when the little girl we had come to see came running in.

We attempted to go up and meet her, and without making eye contact, she ran off in the other direction. It was hard for her foster parent to keep up with her. The caseworker made no attempt to get us seated together or talk about when we would interact more. One of the supervisors came over to us and asked to meet with us for a minute to discuss the girls' case, as she had noticed the interaction between us. We explained how interested we were in caring for the girls, especially now that we had met them and really hit it off. She went into the logistics of the case without getting too specific: the father was protesting termination of rights, the next hearing would be scheduled for January, it was going to be a long process, and so on. Not what I had wanted to hear. I asked questions that she couldn't answer about how the attorneys and the agency were advocating for these girls who had been in the system for three years. She basically just shrugged with the robotic attitude of "it is what it is." This should have been one of my first clues of the cavalier nature and attitude there. The people we encountered within this work environment would have little to no interest in truly helping the kids they were supposed to serve.

As the night continued, the disorganization of the agency became alarmingly more apparent. They had wonderful teen speakers who were going to share their journeys of overcoming foster care, but no one could hear them because the microphone didn't work, and there was no PowerPoint. Most of the foster parents were so busy eating that they were not looking after the children running around wildly and uncontrollably, screaming, taking no notice that there was a presentation that was happening. Disabilities or not, kids need boundaries and expectations. Why was the agency not prepared to accommodate them? It was not a good look and not the type of agency we had signed up for. An hour and a half in, the caseworker still had not come over to have us get to know the little girl we came for.

All the while, we were getting to know the two girls at our table more. They were the best behaved. We were also getting to know their family. I was surprised at the dad. He was not what I expected at all. For starters, he was a lot older. He almost looked the same age as his mother, who sat on the other side of me. They had brought the younger girl a present for her birthday, which had just happened. This meant she was now five. And he doted on each child, ensuring they had what they wanted to eat or drink. I was saddened to hear him making promises to the older child. He told her how he was trying, and in a couple of months, they would all be able to be together again. He also slipped her his cell-phone number. This made me uncomfortable, so I told the caseworker who I knew was on their case.

The longer we sat there, the more disheartened I felt. There was no resolution anytime soon, and I was growing fonder of these girls with every minute that went by. Not only them but also this surreal world where we were all a mixed family and were sitting together enjoying Thanksgiving. My mind raced, thinking that if only someone could explain to this man that we didn't want to cut him out of his daughter's lives, that we would include him and his mother, he would get it and let them be adopted. I was overwhelmed, deflated, and exhausted. We made an abrupt exit. The whole reason we had gone hadn't even come to fruition. We knew it was meant to be, but why did we have to even meet and interact with those girls whom we had wanted since their case had been presented? It just seemed like a cruel test. Were they supposed to be our destiny, and it was just going to take time? I just felt so yucky, and so, like the mature, professional adult that I am with sick days, I talked to my boss about everything that went down, pulled the covers over my head, and called out of work the next day. It was parent-conference day anyway, so I reasoned with myself that it would be fine, and my presence would not be missed too much. I just didn't have the energy. I was so tired of feeling my heartbreak at every unexpected bump in the road.

CHAPTER 6

The Great and Powerful IVF

~⤔

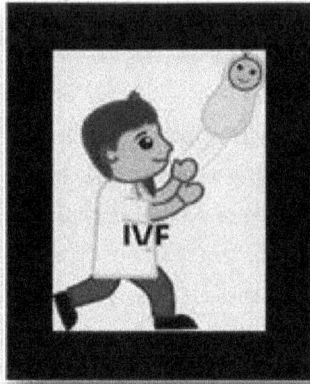

December 2015

ANOTHER MONTH HAD PASSED. IN that interim, I had reached out to the supervisor of my agency to share our concerns. I had launched into a four-paragraph e-mail detailing the frustration we felt. Then, I had conveyed my questions in regard to the case of the girls. I was very professional within the e-mail. Her response indicated that she also did not feel the sense of urgency and advocacy for two little lives who had been in the system for over three years. The follow-up phone call did not make me feel better either. It was all about the system, the procedures in place. Basically, we could continue to wait for this case with little to no hope that it would be resolved anytime soon, or we could hear other cases. We opted for both but said that we wanted to give it until the next court case for the girls to determine if we would hear other cases. We had a home; we wanted to love these girls and give them a good, stable life. Why didn't the lawyers, courts, and agencies involved feel more of a sense of urgency to resolve their case? This was a question I would continue to ask myself more in depth over the following months, never getting an answer that I felt was sufficient.

By the end of December, as a college friend of mine was exploring IVF and a coworker who had extreme difficulty getting pregnant just returned from maternity leave with her beautiful IVF miracle baby, I started to wonder if I had made the right decision by not even considering it. I started to talk to other people who had done it successfully. It was amazing how many people I encountered who had utilized IVF to have babies. All of them had devastating, hopeless, frustrating experiences, and the success of IVF and birth of healthy babies had made the painful memory of it dissipate. Was I cheating myself and Aaron by not even trying this option? When I talked to Aaron about it at length and did more research, we decided it was something we should explore and at least consult with my fertility specialist about.

We had considered doing an IUI: "intrauterine insemination." Think about it like basting a turkey except a more formal medical process where the semen is injected artificially. After we had tried to set this up several times, with Aaron having to do more blood work and playing phone tag between the urologist and fertility center, this process was not moving fast. Furthermore, as my college friend explained (I love her because she had done way more research than me and could share every intricate detail about each procedure), she had done two IUIs already that were not successful. Statistically, as well, they had a much lower success rate than IVF. I then talked to my coworker, who is seriously the kindest, most caring, most beautiful-inside-and-out young woman and teacher I've known. She shared with me how she had struggled with the idea of IVF because of her faith and all the emotions she had experienced as she tried to decide. But at the end of the day, someone had encouraged her just to make a phone call, and it changed her life. She was so heartfelt and grateful. She is the one who inspired me. I made the call to my fertility specialist that day and quickly had an appointment for after the New Year. New Year, new hope: that was what I wished for, trying to say it and put the mantra out into the universe to come true.

So after the holiday break and a nice getaway to Florida where we celebrated the ringing in of the New Year with family, friends, and fireworks, it was time for the appointment. Of course, it was at the end of the day after work. I was so unbelievably nervous, fearing that it would come out that I had another tumor and couldn't even go through with the possibility of IVF. It's funny because when articles, blogs, and so on pop up on Facebook about infertility and you read comments, there are always haters saying things like why don't people just adopt, or why don't they realize that maybe they're not meant to have kids, along with other ignorant things indicating they have never experienced the problem. Like people who are going through infertility have never thought of these things. It plagued me that maybe I wasn't supposed to carry my own child. That maybe my body couldn't handle it. What if I finally did get pregnant through this procedure, and I had a miscarriage? Wouldn't that be worse? What if my uterus hurt the baby in some way, like from a uterine fibroid tumor? Ugh, my mind was spinning, rotating around the negative. Maybe I should just turn around and go home. No, I was going to see this through and at least have the consultation.

My fertility specialist and I had already been through a lot. She had a breathtaking way of bluntly telling the truth, so I knew if it was hopeless, she would be straightforward with me. After the traditional thirty-dollar copay for walking in the door, I was ushered back to my specialist's office. I was strangely comforted by being there. Once we got through the greeting and polite small talk, she asked me how she could help, and I launched into the whole story of what we had been through since the last time I saw her. Visibly touched, she said that I had been through a lot. Then, she went through all the facts and steps for the process, focusing on the fact that she felt like we had really good odds of conceiving through IVF and outlining how it would occur. It was a huge relief. The steps looked like a lot of work, but I had known it was not going to be easy. And it was worth it to be a parent. That's the other thing that people who are ignorant of the struggles of fertility don't understand. Me, as a Christian, spiritual person: If I was not meant to be a parent or have a child, then why was the desire so strong in my heart? God is God and can do anything. If it really wasn't meant to be, then why didn't he just make the desire and will disappear?

Embarking down the IVF route, I had to get another HSG just to make sure that there were no growing tumors. This was another day when I was filled with dread, fear, and anxiety. I had been placed in the same room where I had screamed so loudly in agony a year before. This time, the process was uncomfortable and awkward, as expected, but not painful. I was given a great report. There were no tumors on the horizon. Nothing was preventing me from moving forward on this path. We just had to wait for my next period (another red brick), and then we could get started. I had not been so excited to get a period, I think, in my entire life. Of course, when you want your period to come, it takes its sweet time! Aaron and I began to joke and secretly wish that both things would happen at the same time: we would start going through IVF; then we would get a call that we could foster to adopt the two girls. We would then have three kids. We longed for that possibility.

At the beginning of February, like my period always did, it started with spotting. I was elated and called the fertility center immediately after arriving at work. After about ten minutes on the phone, I had all the necessary appointments booked for the next month to carry out the steps to start IVF. I had gone through the billing office, and they confirmed the breakdown of what my insurance would pay. Pretty much all I would have to pay were the copays (I already knew, as the thirty dollars added up fast), a down payment of $1470, and the necessary costs for my medication to be shipped. Just like that, it was a go for IVF. I felt excited, hopeful, like something was finally happening. My mom was a substitute in my school building at that time, so it wasn't long before I shared the news with her, of course after I had confirmed it with Aaron. She was thrilled!

I got so wrapped up in the activities of my day that I was astonished to return to my office and find a missed call from the placement coordinator from our foster-care agency. My heart skipped a beat. Why was she calling?

Could this be the call that we had wanted for so long? I quickly called her back, and it was confirmed. There was an emergency placement case of two girls who were five and seven. Their parents were not in the picture and hadn't been in years. They were being raised by their grandparents, who could no longer care for them because of medical reasons. The grandparents were terminating their rights the following Monday. The concerns were that they had behaviors, especially the youngest one. She shared how there was no "honeymoon period" with these two girls, which meant they did not act well behaved even for a short time and showed their difficult behaviors right off the bat. Difficult behaviors included the oldest one being "parentified" and the little one along with being hyperactive, to throw tantrums and elope. As I listened to the placement coordinator's explanation, I was amazed at the similarities to the behaviors of the little girl I had become so fond of in my school. ADD, ODD, temper tantrums, and defiance. All in my wheelhouse. When I was told their names, like before with the other case, I immediately looked them up. The two faces I found were the most precious, angelic, happy, and adorable faces I had ever seen. Without confirming it with Aaron, I told our placement coordinator to make the call to express our interest. This case would go fast unless we jumped on it.

Aaron was my direct next call. As I proceeded to fill him in on the girls and all the details, he listened, not interjecting much. I couldn't tell if he was happy or even still alive. When I prompted him for a response, he began to convey some joy and excitement as well. Then, both of our minds started going into shock and overload. Could this be the reason why nothing had worked out before? We were meant to parent these girls? Wasn't it strange how this turn of events happened on the same day I had the IVF appointments all scheduled? What was God trying to tell me? It didn't take long until I felt like I had the answer. Within an hour our placement coordinator had returned our call, stating that a lot of people were interested, but the state had chosen us. The girls would be with us by the end of the week. Wait, like Friday? It was Monday. *Oh my God! Amazing! Oh my God, I'm going to be a mom! Is this really happening? Thank you, God.*

And then—*oh shit, I don't have everything or anything ready for two little girls to feel at home.* So much to do in so little time.

And that was the last part of normalcy within my former life that I knew, because from that point on, there was not a thought, action, feeling, or word I had that did not revolve around these two little lives who changed my world, ideals, and image of being a parent forever.

CHAPTER 7

The Wicked Witch of DSS

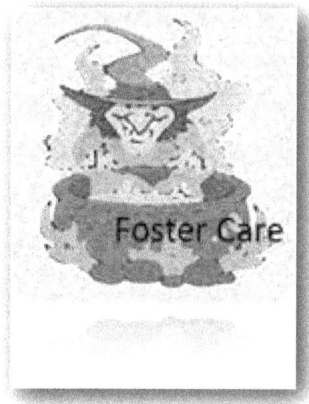

THE COUPLE OF DAYS LEADING up to the girls' arrival into our home were a blur of shopping, cleaning, organizing, and imagining how the house and our life would change. What would they be like? Would our connection be instant, or would it take time? I knew it didn't matter, because no matter what, Aaron and I were intending to adopt them. My school staff had been amazing, and once they heard about the impending arrival of the girls, all the teachers donated stuffed animals, games, toys, and other items that would be needed to make them feel at home in their bedrooms. Little laminated cutout hearts, one with each girl's name on it, were created and placed on their individual bedroom doors.

Silly me, I had thought I could still make the meetings I was scheduled to attend on the Friday of their arrival. On the day, as I was still scrambling to get things as perfect as they could be, I realized that work needed to take a backseat. So I called out of work, heading to Walmart for a last-minute trip of stock-up items. I had never had children at home before, so I wanted to make sure I had everything that could possibly be needed. On the way back from Walmart, I stopped at the grocery store, happily shopping in all the aisles I had never had use for before. After a sizeable amount of money and an abundance of items, I finally felt ready. I was so excited, anticipating their arrival. It was a type of anxiety I had never experienced before. When my phone rang, I knew it was the caseworker to say they were on the way. When I hung up, I turned to Aaron: "Honey, they're on the way." My heart was racing. We both were watching the parking spot outside our house like nosy, snooping neighbors.

When I heard a car pull into the spot, I was out the front door. I saw two adults and two of the cutest little girls I had ever laid eyes on getting out of the car. The littler girl had two pigtails that were bouncing as she walked toward the door. I quickly greeted them and introduced myself. They had two very sad little bags of things, contained in reusable, recycled grocery bags. Our dog quickly met everyone, jumping up excitedly. Aaron introduced himself but had to contain the dog as I got the girls situated. I took them up to their rooms, making small talk to try to help them feel more comfortable. When I showed them that they would each have their own room and explained that everything in there was theirs, I could tell they doubted the words coming out of my mouth. The older one just nodded, while the younger was bouncing around exploring. They quickly slammed their doors, taking in their new surroundings, while I went to talk to the workers who had transported them.

The worker from my agency was also supposed to be arriving. He knew the time. The other workers needed him there to sign off on paperwork. I called—no answer; texted—still no answer. They shared pertinent information with me, such as notes about the girls' care, doctors' names, appointment dates, and dentist's name. We briefly discussed school and agreed that they would transfer to a school closer to our house. After about fifteen minutes, the girls were down in the living room exploring the rest of the house. The dog was bounding after them. All of a sudden, my house had become a chaotic force filled with life. I was still waiting on the caseworker and had to call the placement coordinator to determine his location. Finally, he called me back. I did not want to judge, but he sounded like a moron. Here I was, trying to make small talk with state workers, take care of two foster girls, and get them situated, and he couldn't even show up when he was supposed to. This should have been another red flag about my agency, but I was too excited about these little lives that had now been placed in my care.

It took the worker another forty-five minutes to get there, so long in fact that the workers went out for lunch and came back. The girls were growing restless and, like all children, had no patience for adult conversation. Finally, this guy showed up. He greeted everyone; then, as I was in the midst of getting snacks and other items for the girls, he had the audacity to ask me for a pen. *Seriously, do I look like I have a pen right now?* Thankfully, the worker had one, and after the paperwork was signed off with the promise of temporary guardianship paperwork coming after the court hearing on Monday, it was just Aaron and I with the girls. We wasted no time in putting together the newly acquired car seats and going to the arcade for a late lunch.

When they said there would be no "honeymoon period" with these two, they were not kidding. The little one was already having a fit, bouncing around and not staying in her seat at the restaurant. We spent money on a card for the arcade, and I quickly learned that having them share a card was a nightmare. It didn't take long to burn through fifty dollars. The little one ran off and hid in a closet she shouldn't have been in when we tried to venture back to the table. Yup, they were right about the eloping. Well, at least now we knew and could set boundaries.

We finished our lunch, went to the park near our house, and came back to our new home environment. We settled in and watched TV, all of us piled into our king-size bed. It ended up being way past their bedtime, but hey, they were getting acclimated. Aaron was enjoying giving them piggyback rides, and the girls especially enjoyed bouncing from his shoulders to the posts on our bed, using them as—well, I will say slides. Aaron was getting concerned because it looked like they were using them as poles, but I wasn't going to go there.

As we settled, eating snacks, taking comfort in our new dynamic, I couldn't believe how easy it was with these girls. Yes, they were kids—hyperactive, always wanting something, constantly chatting—but they were now with us, and it felt like they had always been ours. For the afternoon they had called us "Aaron and Chrissie." It had a weird ring. As I tucked the little one in bed that night and read her a story, she asked if she could call me "Mom." When I said yes, she quickly yelled to her sister that they could call us "Mom." It didn't take long for Aaron to hear the word *Mom* being said, and he quizzically asked "Are they calling you 'Mom'?" I told him yes.

"Mom"—hearing two little loves say that to me in their innocent yet needy, childlike tones was a feeling I cannot put into words, but it made my heart fuller than it had ever been. The next day the girls followed suit with calling Aaron "Dad." That first night, after the oldest had fallen asleep, the little one was still having a hard time. We had both nightlights on, had a snack, and had a drink of water, and she still had no luck. At one thirty in the morning, with tears in her eyes, she begged me if she could fall asleep next to me. What was I going to do, say no? How could I say no to that cute little face? She curled up next to me, and it wasn't long until she was off to dreamland. When I awakened at four to find her asleep next to me, I carried her into her room. I didn't want to make this a habit. I felt such a connection to this little girl; there was a part of my soul that just connected with her. She reminded me so much of a kindred spirit to when I was a little girl: cute, feisty, and strong willed.

That first weekend altogether was a blur of activity. We went to McDonald's, the movies, and the park. These girls never tired, and it was almost like they had never done anything, so they wanted to make up for it all at once. Food was a challenge. I had almost bought out the grocery store with kid-like foods. They gobbled up Fruit Roll-Ups, fruit snacks, and Yoo-hoo, but when it came to actually eating anything good for them, they wanted no part of that. We were very thankful when their tablets arrived. We hoped they would keep them occupied. But even with TV and tons of games and toys, they needed our constant attention. The other thing we were realizing about them is that they did not have a very loving sisterly bond. It was almost like the older sister would go out of her way to mess with the younger sister. The first time we tried to take a bath was a battle. It was like they both hated water and forget about brushing their teeth or hair. I knew I was going to have to break out some big-time incentives. Good thing I was a teacher at heart. I had bought crayon paint and bathtub crayons at the advice of some of my teacher-parents at school. Thank God, that got them in the tub.

By Sunday night, Aaron and I were exhausted like we had never been exhausted before. As a childless couple, we had previously enjoyed our week-ends—sleeping in, relaxing, and actually watching adult shows or even any show. After being initiated with these two at ages five and seven, we had no peace and were constantly entertaining them. But we were parents, and we loved them. After all, school was the next day. Never in my life had I been so thankful for school. We had decided we would transport them to their old school for one last day so they could get their things and say good-bye to their teachers and friends. Of course, the little one being in pre-K meant she only had an afternoon program. Aaron and I had taken off work for a couple of days to get the girls acclimated. We were excited to have a couple of hours to ourselves once they were in school to catch our breath and touch base, something we hadn't been able to do all weekend.

I got up early, packed the older girl's lunch, wrote a cute little note like my mom had always done for me, and woke her up. She was very compliant, quickly getting dressed and gathering her things. I attempted to chat on the car ride over, but she was very sullen. I couldn't tell if it was because she was sad to leave her school or because we just hadn't really connected yet. She was hard to read. I waited in my car and watched her go in, feeling proud that I had gotten a child off to school as a mom. It had taken twenty minutes to drive there and twenty minutes back, a drive we would have to do again to take the little one to pre-K at twelve thirty. I was thankful when I got home that the little one was asleep.

It wasn't an hour later though that my phone rang, and it was the school. We had to come get the older one because she had head lice. Lice? What, really? Ugh. When the workers had dropped her off, they said that she had *had* lice and needed to be treated within seven to ten days. They didn't say anything about active lice. All my years as a teacher and educator, I had never dealt with it in my home. Welcome to parenthood? We quickly got the little one together and all made the trek back to their school. The nurse was kind; she showed us where the lice were in her head and explained how we needed to administer the treatment and what to do. She also shared that this had been a *chronic* problem all year. That would have been nice to know when the workers dropped off the girls.

The little one was also checked out. Thankfully, she did not have any lice, so she would be able to go to school, but it was not yet time. So we headed to the playground, had a little snack, and waited for the pre-K class to open. I walked her up to the door, meeting the teacher and explaining the new situation. I immediately did not like the teacher, as I could tell she had judged the little one, writing her off as a problem child. The nurse, who was kind, had also commented to me about the little one's behaviors. I watched as the little one began to act different in the classroom, running off, not following the rules. Yes, she had some incidents over the weekend, but her behaviors were not within the character I had observed. I made a note in my mind to talk with her about it later. We traveled back home with the older one in tow. Looked like there would be no quiet or time to regroup today. Again, I thanked God that I worked in a school and had the best nurse in the entire county. I got her instructions along with those of other parents, and we did the shampoo, combed it out, and instituted a mayonnaise head on the older one, much to her dismay. It smelled disgusting, but she took it like a champ, even sleeping with the mayonnaise head overnight.

I was a little astonished that no workers had really checked in. Sure, our agency worker had called to check in the day after the girls were dropped off, but after we were handed the court paperwork and the state agency worker transferred over, there had been no contact. I had reached out to our agency to try to get the new worker's phone number, but of course, it had been over forty-eight hours, and he hadn't had any luck. The next endeavor was getting the girls transferred and enrolled in the school closest to us. I finally understood what all parents go through to register their students. The secretaries were curt when I was trying to navigate the process over the phone. After calls to resource people within the county, I was elated that they were able to get the little one into the pre-K program at the school. It had been a lot of runaround. Gathering up all the bills, the mortgage, and the completed registration forms, I headed to the new school to try to get them enrolled. It was a task. The only thing we needed now was the state worker to do her part. Oh, if only I could get in touch with her. I finally had gotten her number myself from the prior state worker and had left a couple of messages. I couldn't believe they could just drop kids off like this with little to no follow-up about the transition. We'd had them now for four days. I explained the lice situation to the secretaries and knew we would need to touch base with the nurse when the girls were slated to arrive. It was interesting, the stigma I had gotten when registering the girls and explaining that they were in foster care. The oldest secretary had asked, "Oh, do you foster a lot?" Her demeanor changed when I explained that we did not and we were fostering them to adopt.

I finally heard from the state worker that afternoon. She said she had no idea about the lice and had not gotten any of my messages. Really? We were off to a great start. Anyway, she seemed pleasant enough on the phone and said that she would sign off on her part of the paperwork to get them enrolled in school. I wanted to get them there as soon as possible to get them into a routine. I was thankful that my boss and work environment were letting me be flexible. Not knowing the reality of parenthood, I had not prepared to be so engrossed with things. I felt like the girls were literally all I could focus on, and I was drowning in even keeping up with work e-mail.

Finally, it was the day to take them to school. We knew we would have to get them checked out by the nurse. I prayed those disgusting lice were gone. As we were getting out of the car to go into school, we realized the older one had sneaked on colored lip gloss. She looked ridiculous, but it made her feel beautiful and comfortable, so what were we going to do at that point? As I checked into the office, Aaron made his way with the girls to the nurse. We were both dressed down in casual attire, so it wasn't evident that we both held positions in the same educational system. The minute I walked into the nurse's office, I could tell it was not going well. Aaron had a disgusted look on his face, and it didn't take me long to see why. This nurse's attitude was ridiculous. She was speaking in a tone that was almost scolding us, scoffing at the active lice she supposedly found in both girls' heads. They could not come to school, because they had active lice. Of course, she didn't bother pulling them out of the girls' heads. She went through the same step of directions the other nurse had told us. When we explained that the little one had been all clear just a couple of days earlier, she again scoffed. I know my nurse at my school wouldn't act like this toward parents or students. Who did this chick think she was? It really felt like she was judging us and the girls because they were in "foster care."

I hate having to throw around my position title, but I knew it would come up with this chick. Aaron being Aaron, of course, had not said anything to her, but he relayed to me in the car that her first comment when they went in the office was, "Oh, she's wearing lipstick," almost rolling her eyes as she said it, indicating that we were the worst parents alive. To make matters worse, we still hadn't had one second of peace because of these damn lice keeping the girls out of school. We had bagged all the pillows and stuffed animals, vacuumed, changed the sheets, and so on. Ugh! I wished for boys at that moment so we could just shave their heads and be done.

My nurse, sympathetic to our plight and disgusted by the way the other nurse had spoken to us, told me about this magical place called a lice clinic. Boom, no more of me trying to wrangle with the damn shampoo and comb. The girls immediately had appointments. I had to go into work for at least a little while, so Aaron took them. It wasn't long though until he was on the phone. The little one needed my prompting to behave long enough to get the treatment. It cost $175 for each girl. Ouch, my wallet was taking a hit since we got kids. But we got a thirty-day guarantee and a certificate. Suck on that, nurse!

The day of this treatment aligned with the first visit we would have with the girls' paternal grandparents, the ones who had taken care of them for over two years. I was a nervous wreck. I had told Aaron to get their hair washed after the appointment, but the oil that was used for the lice treatment stuck to their heads like glue. There was no way to rectify that beforehand, as traveling to the visit was going to take at least twenty-five minutes, so I just hoped the grandparents would understand. I wondered what they would be like and if they would like us. I had tried to prep the girls for what to expect, but really, I had no idea myself. The worker had said we would have an "icebreaker," whatever the hell that meant, with just the grandparents and us at first. Then, they would visit with the girls for an hour. On the way there, I asked the girls if they thought their grandparents would like us, and the little one said, "Of course, they will love you." It gave me some relief.

We showed up at what I thought was the right place. It's not like there had been explicit directions, just a text message with the name of the place. We were clearly on the wrong side, but a kind worker took pity on us as we sat in the play area attempting to call our worker. The person assisting us was clearly from a different department and rolled her eyes at the lack of clarification and availability of the state worker. It was evident these two departments had issues. When I finally got the worker on the phone, she seemed exasperated that I had not known where to go. Yeah, like we had visited DSS a whole lot before this? Um, no. As difficult as it obviously was for her to go a bit out of her way, she walked the corridor between the two buildings and brought us through what seemed like a long maze of hallways filled with cubicles to the appropriate area. She then shared that these two other workers were going to take the girls to Petco while we met with the grandparents. The girls immediately freaked out. They did not want to leave our sides, and I had not prepared them for that. We calmed them down as best we could.

It was finally time to meet the grandparents. When Aaron and I were introduced to them, it was almost as if my whole soul had a collective sigh of relief. They were really cool and kind people. Almost immediately, we were going back and forth in conversation, excited to get to know one another as fellow caregivers for two amazing little girls. When the worker finally interrupted the conversation, she stunned us all by saying the plan was for "reunification" with their birth parents. Wait a minute; we were a pre-adoptive resource? Hadn't the grandparents had rights that were terminated? I was very confused and attempted to set her straight, explaining that our agency should have told them we were in this for adoption. She reiterated that the plan initially was always for reunification. The grandparents launched into their knowledge about the birth parents, how they were both addicted to heroin, and the girls would never have happy, healthy lives with them. They shared that they were fine with us adopting them, because they wanted the girls to have a great life. It was an interesting turn of events, to say the least, and I didn't quite know what to make of it.

We were then ushered into a room with a two-way mirror. It was a very sad playroom with dirty toys and sad-looking seating options. The grandparents, enjoying our company, had invited us in to the visit with them to play with the girls. It was evident from their interactions with them that they loved the girls. They were filling us in on some vital family history when the worker interrupted, stating that we should make sure we were talking about things that were appropriate. Seriously? This was appropriate. We were trying to understand where they came from. It was the first time I felt like a criminal being observed and reprimanded by the state, but it wouldn't be the last time I felt like that within the process.

The worker confirmed that she could still come over that night to do the home visit. Although I was exhausted, I confirmed that it was fine. Aaron had to rush off to night class, so it would just be me, the worker, and the girls. When we got home, the girls began their norm of running around hyperactively, needing constant attention. It was very difficult to carry on a conversation. The worker explained again that the plan was for reunification. Puzzled, I asked my clarifying questions, focusing on one in particular: "You're not going to actually return them to drug addicts, right?" She looked at me quizzically, like she didn't understand what was wrong with that proposition. I would need to get in touch with my agency to find out what the hell was going on. This was not what we signed up for. She also explained that the girls had other family members who wanted to visit with them, and she would be in touch to set up those visits. Great? I explained that we didn't want to keep them from visiting with anyone, and I really meant that, but I had no idea what I was in for or the toll the visits were about to take on the girls.

The rest of this chapter will highlight behavior logs and a similar timeline of events that would later be submitted to one of the top people in charge of the state department, as these are the most pertinent pieces of information I can use to convey what we all went through in just trying to love two little girls and give them a permanent home. Names are not listed, and items have been paraphrased at times to honor confidentiality.

> February 23, 2016: The state worker notifies us via text that she is working on setting up a visit with maternal grandmother for February 29, 2016, at 4:30 p.m. She says, "It will be four thirty at DSS. We can meet in the front lobby where the Drumcastle sign is. Closest to the shopping center. Yes, you can meet the grandmother, and we can discuss how often visits will be moving forward."
>
> February 24, 2016: Therapy session with state worker in attendance. The foster parent asks about visitation with the biological mom. **The therapist shares verbal recommendations for a slow transition to visitation with Mom. The state worker says' that visitation has not yet been set up with the biological mother and to put the recommendations in writing for the court.**

As an educator who was certified in special education and an IEP facilitator, I stupidly believed that the foster-care system would put the same amount of weight on recommendations from the therapist as a school would when trying to help a child be successful. So when the little one's therapist had recommended that possible visits with Mom occur in a slow transition if at all, I believed that would happen. Always wanting to know whom I was dealing with, I of course had looked up their mom in the court system. She was convicted of confinement and second-degree child abuse. I knew that she had recently been released from prison and had transitioned into a halfway house, as it was public record. I did speak to the state worker in regard to that, and she assured me that no visitation or communication with the mother had yet occurred. I breathed a sigh of relief. The girls had been with their grandparents for almost two years. Maybe there was a chance she wouldn't want them back. And if she did, surely once she met us and saw the life we wanted to give them, she would want them to be well provided for, right? It was hard for me to comprehend a mother who wouldn't want her kids to have the world if it was something she could not provide them.

When it came time for another visit, this time with the girls' other grand-mother, I had wanted to meet her because we had formed such a great bond with the paternal grandparents. And because I naively thought that if she met us and saw how much we loved the girls, as well as how happy they were, she would support them living with us. The experience with the paternal grand-parents had gone so well that I was definitely not prepared for the hostile visit with this person that was about to take place.

February 29, 2016: Text from the state worker at 9:14 a.m.: "I have a meeting at five o'clock, and I won't be able to supervise the visit, so my coworker will supervise, but she will meet you in the lobby on the Drumcastle side of the building."

Great, I was already nervous, and now the worker we knew wasn't even going to be the one supervising. As we made the trip to DSS, I asked the girls if Mom-Mom would like us. This time, the little one hesitated to answer me. The older one said that she would, but I could sense from the little one that we were in for a rude awakening. We checked in with the security room and headed to the waiting area. I saw an older lady with tattoos walk in, and the security guard pointed our way. I greeted her politely as the girls ran up to give her hugs. Our worker and the worker who would be supervising came out after that and took us to the play area, telling the girls not to touch anything. Um, seriously, they're kids, and they're quite hyperactive. Good luck with that! We sat down with Mom-Mom, who immediately started interrogating us, making her disgust known that we had them transferred to a new school and that she could no longer interact with them. She asked about phone calls and when the girls would visit with their mother. I was shocked at her hostility toward us. I looked to the supervising state worker for some answers or any indication that she was going to respond, but she remained quiet. I simply deferred and told her she would have to discuss the regulations with their caseworker. Then, I got Aaron and me out of there. Ugh, that was rough and not what I had expected! I felt like a criminal. Like we were doing something wrong by trying to care for these girls. Hadn't visitation been explained to her? Why did our state worker for the girls not prepare us for that? It was definitely something I was going to have to follow up with her about.

> February 29, 2016: Visit with Mom-Mom occurred. As we reentered the building to pick the girls up, we were summoned back to the observation room by the security guard. The worker supervising asked us if the girls' behavior was typical. They were running around uncontrollably while Mom-Mom was texting on her phone. During this time span, the little one was locked in a cabinet multiple times by her sister. Her sister took the wooden rocking chair and wedged it against the cabinet so the little one could not get out. The supervising worker told us to calm down when we got upset watching this. It was explained to her that the little one had issues with confinement and this would re-traumatize her. Again, we were told to "calm down."

I really felt like I was being "punked" or in a really bad movie. I cannot convey to you the horror I felt as I witnessed the girls' behavior on the other side of the two-way mirror. They were running around like animals, hopping on things. When the older one pushed the younger one into the cabinet and closed the door, then trying to get a wooden rocking chair in order to wedge it to confine her in there, while Mom-Mom texted away on her phone not paying one bit of attention, I thought I was going to jump through the window. I knew the ramifications of this with the diagnosis of PTSD: the night terrors this would raise, the dissociation, and the tantrums later. Why in the hell was this worker allowing this to continue, and was she fucking serious to calm down? We had been interrupted by our state worker due to a damn conversation, but this was allowed to continue. Seriously? I was livid, and for anyone who knows me, that is always evident on my face and with my demeanor. As the visit ended, the worker begged me not to say anything. I literally wanted to punch Mom-Mom in the face. How could she allow them to treat one another like that? All of our rules and expectations went out the window. I reminded myself that I was not sixteen again and was a professional, gathered myself, and went to the girls as they ran up and hugged us. I was very thankful the little one pulled me away, having to immediately use the bathroom, so I did not have to interact with Mom-Mom. On our way out though, she of course got a selfie to show their biological mom. I had so many emotions running through me: anger, disgust, horror, and shock. All I wanted to do was get them out of there and go home. I felt like I was going to throw up. But I turned it off to ensure the girls were OK. My feelings were tabled as we transitioned them out, had a car picnic of pizza, and made our way home. Being a parent is a lot like being an assistant principal: everyone else's wants and needs come before your own, no matter how you are feeling or what may be going on personally for you.

Text to the state worker from us at 5:38 p.m.: "During the visit, the little one was locked in a cabinet multiple times by her sister with the worker observing, while the girls were with Mom-Mom. This is very concerning to us."

Response text: "OK I will follow up with the worker and make the therapy program aware of these acting-out behaviors so they can get an intake scheduled as soon as possible."

Our response: "Mom-Mom seemed very confused about the process of visitation, directed some anger our way, and shared that her daughter was out of jail and wanted to know when she was going to get visitation. This visit may cause serious regression for the little one's PTSD as she was confined to dark spaces often by her mother and Mom-Mom in this case did nothing to stop it. Her diagnosis was officially changed to PTSD on Friday by her therapist."

State worker's response text: "I will speak with my supervisor about this tomorrow. I also have concerns about these behaviors during visits."

Ours: "Great, thank you! It was just so hard to watch. We love both of them so much and hate seeing them regress."

State worker: "I'm glad we were able to see the lack of supervision on Mom-Mom's behalf, so this makes me question further visits with her."

February 29, 2016: Evening e-mail communication occurred regarding the incident at the visit informing the therapist as well as our agency.

When we shared what happened that evening, I was amazed at our agency's worker's lack of shock. He simply dismissed the behaviors as ones that all foster kids do, minimalizing our feelings. Although the state worker had seemed equally upset with the events, her e-mails also reiterated the same level of complacency, like we were the ones overreacting. I felt like I was going insane. Thankfully, the therapist called the next morning. She agreed that it was retraumatizing, making me feel like we were the ones keeping the girls' best interests at hand.

This whole thing was really taking a toll on me. I was too emotionally invested, and all the appointments, along with the stress of visits and dealing with multiple workers, put me on edge. I knew I needed to take leave from work. Thankfully, I had the days and an understanding boss. I informed her that I was taking the family leave that I was due for having foster girls. It was even more awesome because my mom, who had been long-term subbing at my school, would be able to take my place as the assistant principal in the interim. Now that I didn't have to feel guilty about work, I could put all my focus on the girls. The little one was relieved she would no longer have to go to daycare in the morning prior to pre-K. Our wallet was also relieved, as even though we were going to the cheapest yet most trustworthy daycare, it was still $150 a week. Not to mention, we wouldn't get our first check for them until the end of March. Geez, how do parents do it? Our weekly grocery bill had expanded to over $300, let alone the day-to-day upkeep of activities, along with school supplies, clothes, and shoes. OK, so I was spoiling them a lot, but they were now my babies. They would want for nothing.

Additionally, I was having to communicate with so many people—the state worker, our worker, the therapist, the psychiatrist, the alliance worker, and so on. I had to send weekly logs to our worker, and personally I also kept behavioral logs. They were really in-depth because I didn't know what would be important and what wouldn't, especially for the little one's therapy. Along with that, we were giving daily points to both of them on my phone app that aligned with their success charts. I also had calm-down tents, a vibe mitt for sensory stimulation, and many other things I had found on NationalAutismResources. com. Although the little one did not have any form of autism, I found that she responded similarly to sensory materials. I also had bulletin boards that emulated positive characteristics, such as responsibility, cooperation, and how to deal with anger, hung on every viable wall surface. The girls each had their visual daily routine and responsibility charts as well, along with their button-incentive mason jars, where we had them deposit buttons that represented the number on their success charts. We did this each night.

> March 3, 2016: We sent an e-mail communication requesting a meeting to discuss what occurred at the visit with the state worker, the worker that had supervised the visit, and her boss along with our agency to discuss this event and future guidelines for visits along with our role in these visits. Also in this e-mail was: **"I also believe that the therapist has the documentation requested by you for the courts."**

State workers' e-mail response in regard to visitation:

1. Visits with the parental grandparents will be biweekly and I am attempting to arrange another supervised visit at DSS with them on Friday, March 11, 2016, from 4:30 p.m. to 5:30 p.m.
   - If this visit goes well and there are no concerns with them being in the community with the girls, these biweekly visits can be unsupervised and arranged between the foster parents and grandparents.
2. Visits with "Mom-Mom" will be monthly and will be supervised at DSS. I think it would be easiest if we just arrange for the same day each month. For instance, the third Tuesday of each month is something that would likely work for my schedule.

After setting up a meeting but having the state and our agency respond like we were "overreacting," even though the therapist had confirmed it was in fact re-traumatization, I had had enough and decided it was time to meet with an attorney. Thankfully, through my position and union at my job, I am entitled to a free consultation.

The day of my consultation, I was really anxious. I hoped there was a way for them to help me but knew it was daunting, as foster parents often do not have any rights under the legal system. Also, it was really early on in the case. The office was located right near my church, which gave me some relief. It was also the week of Aaron's birthday, so if the girls got off the bus and followed directions, we were going to go out as a family to a really nice dinner at a Japanese steak house. The attorney's office was beautiful and really stood out, with the decor like in one of the offices you see on a legal show like *Boston Legal*. In my senior year of college, I took a law course for my minor and almost switched my whole track to become a family-law attorney. Now, I was wishing I had and that I had the expertise to be able to help the situation.

The attorney I met with seemed very distinguished and well put together. After greetings and small talk, I launched into the story and all the events that had occurred. Although through her experiences she was not shocked at what she heard, she was touched with empathy at our plight, explaining how we were not the "typical" parents in the foster-care system. She explained the process and the timeline and recommended that we follow up with the girls' attorney, which was probably the only recourse we had at that time. She even gave me her private cell-phone number and offered to go to their court hearing with me in July just to explain what was occurring. The outcome was what I thought it would be: there was nothing she could do to help us at that time, but I felt good that I had such a great resource whom I could touch base with as we continued this process. She did caution me to follow the guidelines that the state was setting, as they could take the girls at any time if they so wished.

As I drove off, I heard from our agency. We had the date and time of the meeting set with the state worker and her supervisor to discuss the "re-trauma-tization." Good. I was hoping we could all come to a combined consensus of what would be in the best interests of the girls. Surely when the supervisor met us and saw our intentions, she would be sympathetic to our plight and would intervene for the girls. Again, with my naïveté and lack of understanding of the system, I had no idea what we were getting into. I got home and picked up the girls and Aaron, and we went and had an enjoyable family dinner at the Japanese steak house. The older one, becoming a connoisseur of food and loving high-quality experiences, enjoyed every second. The little one only wanted ice cream, which I indulged her in, trying to get her to sit peacefully for the dinner. Of course, when she realized it was fried, she wanted no part of it. Thankfully, the food show entertained her, and we ended up being the only ones in the restaurant. It was a great night.

March 11, 2016: Visit at DSS with paternal grandparents. They offered for us to stay during their visit. We looked to the state worker for advice. She did not offer any advice one way or another. We left. When we returned and asked about unsupervised visits in the future, we were told every two weeks and in the community. No other recommendations, expectations, or guidelines were given in regard to unsupervised visitation.

March 15, 2016: Meeting occurred to discuss the incident with our agency, the state worker, and her supervisor. We were informed that it was never the intent to retraumatize a child at the state. We discussed the little one's updated diagnosis of PTSD and the therapist's recommendation. They shared that the only room available at the time of the visit was in transition, and the room was being changed over to get new furniture. The girls had been told not to touch any of the toys during the visit, which they shared was an unrealistic expectation. The cabinet has since been moved out of the room. It also was shared that it was the worker's first supervised visit. We should not have been called back by security. We shared that we preferred to not see any of the visitations occur or to be called back from this point forward. The timeline of visitation was discussed in regard to the biological mom as well as how we were a pre-adoptive resource. We were told that visits with the biological mom would not be occurring anytime soon, and when they did, it would be a gradual transition.

I ended up really liking the state worker's supervisor. She seemed shocked that our agency would have given us this case, which gave me pause about the people we had signed up with, but overall she was warm toward us. It was evident that she had been in the system a long time. She shared that they always said they wanted "people" like us, but she wanted to caution us from loving them too much, as she didn't want to see us get hurt. I didn't know how to do that. I already loved them and thought of them as my own. How could I put the brakes on that? When we discussed their biological mother, I asked what she was like. I had so many images in my mind, and I even had dreams that I would meet her, we would talk, and she would agree to let us adopt them once she knew we would love them and give them a better life. That image shattered when the state worker said she met girls' biological mom once in court, and the mother literally yelled out wishing everyone in the court dead. What do you say to that? For once, I was speechless. When they assured us that visitation would not happen anytime soon, I was relieved but felt the sinking feeling in my stomach return, growing stronger with each passing week.

> March 21, 2016: During a weekly text with paternal grandparents, we are told by them that we have a visit with Mom-Mom the next day. In review of previous e-mails from the worker, we were told that visits would be the last Tuesday of the month. This does not fall in line with what was outlined. When we e-mail the worker for clarification, she calls the next morning, shares she forgot about the month having five weeks, and asks us if we are able to attend as she already set up the visitation with Mom-Mom.

Fucking seriously, we have to see and interact with this woman again? Spring break was starting that weekend, and I had been excitedly getting the girls' clothes, suitcases, and other items ready. We were taking them to Florida to stay at my mom's condo. It would be their first time on a plane and to Florida. It was also Easter weekend and our first Easter together, so I was running around trying to get the cutest baskets, things to dye Easter eggs, and photos set up with the Easter bunny. I was really also looking forward to getting away from it all and having family time where we could just relax without having to rush off to school, an appointment, or a visit. Between our worker, the state worker, and the other community worker assigned through a separate company, there were constantly people at our house or people we needed to follow up with. The weekly logs that we were required to send took me hours to compile. Even though I was off from work, it really felt like I had a full-time job with the documentation, not to mention just doing the typical chores of a stay-at-home mom. I just felt sick at the idea of having to interact again. But of course, I agreed, we made the appointment, and I somehow that day resolved to be the bigger person. I was a Christian after all. Love the unlovely; overcome evil with good, right? It was definitely easier said than done, but I decided to make her a photo album nonetheless.

March 22, 2016: Visit with Mom-Mom. We give her a book made by Walgreens Photo of updated pictures of the girls.

The state worker had offered to pick the girls up and drive them to this visit. I was relieved that our interaction would only be one sided and that we didn't have to make two trips. Because of the upcoming Florida trip, I tried to remain as relaxed as I could. The state worker looked shocked when I handed her the book that I had made for Mom-Mom. As we picked up the girls, they were talking about Florida, and all Mom-Mom could say was how she had family in Florida and would take them when the girls returned to their mother. I rolled my eyes on the inside.

Below are snapshots of one of the success charts, along with the behavioral data I collected for the first six weeks. It was a full-time job. There was so much to each child, so many emotions, and so much trauma. It was heart-breaking to hear, let alone reread and document. But I wanted to ensure that they would get the proper care and treatment from all the medical professionals working with them, so I documented away. I wanted you as the reader to truly understand and take in the types of things the girls were saying and doing every day as this was such a trying time of determining how to best support them.

Subject	I managed my emotions by using appropriate calm down strategies and was able to identify how I was feeling and why.	I kept my hands, feet and body to myself at all times AND did not hurt myself on purpose in any way.	Comments
Morning	☺ ☺ ☺	☺ ☺ ☺	
Morning	☺ ☺ ☺	☺ ☺ ☺	
Afternoon	☺ ☺ ☺	☺ ☺ ☺	
Afternoon	☺ ☺ ☺	☺ ☺ ☺	
Afternoon	☺ ☺ ☺	☺ ☺ ☺	
Night	☺ ☺ ☺	☺ ☺ ☺	
Night	☺ ☺ ☺	☺ ☺ ☺	
Night	☺ ☺ ☺	☺ ☺ ☺	

Reward Choices	Amount	Consequences
Can redeem for activity or bank for a larger reward	6-13	Reflection Sheet
	0-6	Loss of 10 minutes phone/iPad/Kindle Time

Compiled Behavior Data

The Little One

Week 1

February 14: Peed in Play-Doh cup while Mom was at youth group; had a meltdown where she was screaming and throwing things. Said it was because her sister wasn't sharing the Wii. (Fourth pee incident; all other times she said she couldn't make it to the bathroom.)

February 15: Lost point money because of inappropriate Amazon purchase (Acting like a demon; said Mom had a demon baby. Wanted to watch Freddy Krueger. When she saw a black man in a music video, she shared he looked like her dad—he was cute, and she liked black boys better.)

February 16:

Rough evening. Created a calm-down spot in the hamper. Lots of meltdowns in the evening. Extreme difficulty falling asleep even with melatonin. Lied about mine craft. When caught, escalated into full meltdown with screams, and tears to a level that had not been yet observed. Trigger to flashback possibly. Calmed down in the room. When asked about it, she shared we could "delete her." It was explained that, no matter how she acted, we would never delete her.

February 17: Kept repeating Daddy has an ex-girlfriend and insisting Daddy and Mommy aren't married.

February 18: Very rough evening: melted down and hit the foster mom and sister; displayed self-injurious behavior such as banging her head on the ground while lying and screaming; yelled, "I don't want to talk about it." Major meltdown lasted about fifteen minutes in duration.

February 19: While eating her snack, she peed through her dress, all over the chair and floor. When asked why and calmly told this was not OK and she needed to ask, she ran up to her room screaming and banging objects.

February 20: More frequent hitting. Poured milk and wiped hands on Mom, and then would run away and break down even when Mom said she wasn't mad. Drew on the closet door when upset about her sister's conversation about biological parents. Refused to clean up toys; periodically broke down to avoid clean up; shut herself in the calm-down tent. Asked Mom to go with her to the bathroom saying she's afraid.

February 21: Great day! Used a minion to be in the bathroom to help allevi-ate her fear. At 7:30 p.m. had a meltdown; calmed down for a minute and then poured chocolate milk on the foster dad and bed sheets. Then completely broke down, put shorts on her head, yelled no, and would not look at the foster mom but indicated she did not want Mom to leave (fifteen minutes in duration). Finally took off shorts and was able to do deep breathing and talk through it; shared she thought parents were mad.

Week 2

February 22: Good day with the routine; broke down around 7:30 p.m. (crying, screaming, and refusal to get dressed; lasted about ten minutes before calming and taking redirection; seems to happen when tired).

February 23: Great day; stuffed up in the morning and upset. Calmed, got dressed, and went to daycare and school. Made cookies with Mom. Great report from school! Minor meltdown around 8:00 p.m. when medicine spilled; took off nightgown, refused to get dressed, and cried for five minutes.

February 24: Extremely difficult day/night managing emotions. Didn't want homemade lasagna at dinner (cried, screamed, and ran to her room; this happened twice for about five minutes each). Came down, took clothes off stuffed cat in the hat toy, and then stripped down and attempted to put those clothes on. In the bathtub she refused to rinse shampoo out of her hair, screamed when the foster parent attempted stating she was afraid, lasted three minutes with screaming/crying, and finally let the foster mom rinse it out in the sink.

*When asked about the breakdown at the KKI visit, she shared she melted down because she had fought with Grandmother over the use of her phone there. The foster mom assured her that she could talk to her in those moments about how she was feeling.

February 25: Good day; meltdown at 8:30 p.m. (asked to use the Vicks vapor rub, didn't use it properly, and said it burned; screamed, cried, and ran out of room when Mom offered wet cloth; was able to use words to express feelings within one to two minutes).

February 26: Rough drop off at daycare: called Mom, needed to say good-bye and hug Dad multiple times, and then when daycare worker tried to intervene, she hit her with a stuffed animal on the head screaming, "Let me go." Meltdown occurred when she saw the dinner she ordered and didn't like it. The foster mom had talked to her about the daycare incident on the ride back home from bowling. In the car she stated that she did wrong by hitting and deserved the time-out at daycare. Amid the breakdown, she wanted to call her daycare provider to apologize and then said her provider was mean to her and she didn't deserve the consequence. Stripped off clothes and got under the covers—thirteen minute duration. She was asleep soon after the breakdown.

February 27: Great day! Interacted well with a student with autism who came over to play at the park. Only breakdown occurred at 8:35 p.m. when going to bed (for some reason wanted to go to the attic and pouted when she couldn't even after it was explained why it was unsafe up there). Has continued to need a foster parent to go with her to the bathroom.

February 28: Was able to verbalize she was upset when her sister started talking about her mom on the ride to church. Still requesting the foster mom to go to the bathroom with her. (She is sharing more that it's because she's afraid of her real mom locking her in the bathroom.) Great at Sunday school. Upset on the ride home with the food choice—again was able to verbalize how she was feeling. Good time outside with making S'mores in the fire pit, started to disengage during family movie time, threw water on her sister during tub time, and then got water all over the dog. This triggered a meltdown that included refusal to get out of the tub. Once out of the tub, refused to get dressed and kicked Dad; when it was shared that it hurt, she screamed, ran into her room, and banged on the doors. When the door was closed so she could calm down, she started to yell, "I hate this family." This continued for about ten minutes. When the foster mom came in, she was under the covers still topless. When eye contact was made, she smiled but hid under her puppy bear. The foster mom asked if she was ready to get dressed. She said yes, got out from under the covers for Mom to hug her, and then very aggressively started hugging, kissing Mom, and trying to look down her shirt. Mom redirected her and told her that was inappropriate as that was a private area. She kept tugging at the shirt and then got distracted by putting play makeup on her doll and the texture of the lipstick. After seven minutes she came downstairs. Meltdown started again when prompted to go upstairs for bedtime, threw Go-Gurt on wall, and did clean it up and apologize. Got dressed, lay with Mom and Sister, and was asleep fifteen minutes later. (Noticing a pattern of her doing something wrong, running away, screaming and banging like she is trying to punish herself, and she feels ashamed; also noticing more aggressive hugging, kissing, and tackling occurring even when asked to stop. The day before she tried to pull Dad's pants down thinking it was funny.)

Triggers appear to be food and being tired.

Week 3

February 29: On the ride to the visit, she shared that she did not want to be left alone with Mom-Mom. A nonverbal cue was worked out with the little one, the foster parents, and DSS. Almost immediately after seeing Mom-Mom, serious regression occurred. She reverted to behavior of a toddler: running around, jumping on things, tearing things up, having difficulty responding to directions, crying, unable to use words to express feelings, and so on. A lot of cuddling, reinforcement of expectations, and comfort and basic needs: food and shelter was focused on for the rest of the evening.

March 1: Serious regression this afternoon: attempted to eat plastic and foam from paper plates, running around without a clear purpose, difficulty responding to directions, and was asleep by 7:25 p.m. (This has never happened since she's been with us.)

March 2: Came home early from school as she didn't feel well; lost five points for not following directions. Around 6:00 p.m. power struggle occurred when she refused to give back Mom's cell phone. She was asked twice and said no. Points were taken away, and she said that was fine. The phone was taken out of her hand by Dad. She then began to cry—screaming multiple times, "I hate you, Dad." Followed by stomping upstairs, screaming, "I miss Grandmother." Both parents shared they would give her time to calm down and then talk. Took five minutes to calm down, and then she was able to articulate how she was feeling, listen to how parents were feeling, and reenact what the appropriate response should have been when the phone was requested. All apologized, and she and parents said they loved one another multiple times. Mom reinforced no matter what she said or did that they would love her, that it was OK to miss her grandmother, and that we could text her soon.

*Since Monday she has been taking her shirt off and wrapping in a blanket shortly after snack/dinner, seeming to need the soothing sensation of the blanket on her skin. She does not like to put a shirt on for one to three hours when she feels this way, even after bath time.

Week 4

March 7: Very hyperactive from time home after school: with Dad when trying to get in a spot to watch TV repeatedly, kicked her sister in the head, and was unable to articulate why. Started to meltdown at 8:30 p.m. when the tablet got unplugged and screamed, "I hate you." She was able to be redirected (after screaming this, she hides her face and doesn't want to make eye contact) ten minutes.

March 8: Rough drop off at daycare; hit Dad, continual screaming of "I hate you"; around 7:00 p.m. put water and fruity pebbles on the dog; and was given time-out. Took the five minute time-out in her room without argument and was able to talk afterward sharing that she thought the dog wanted to be dressed up. Good talk occurred, she understood why the behavior was wrong, and she was able to move on.

March 9: Great day: no meltdowns. Cried out in the middle of the night around eleven o'clock (three times); sore throat and disoriented.

March 10: Awesome day: no meltdowns. Cried out in sleep around 10:30 p.m., screaming, "I want my ballie." Once she was given a ball, she took it and fell back to sleep. At 1:00 a.m. cried out, "Mommy"—had a bad dream about leprechauns. Up until 3:30 a.m. crying out intermittently for Mommy or Daddy, "My tummy hurts."

March 11: Slept until 11:00 a.m. and no recollection of waking up; good day.

March 12: Rough day: a lot of tears, easily upset, and new environment at Aaron's parents' house.

March 13: Good day: at restaurant had difficulty not running in the arcade at dinner—overstimulated.

Week 5

March 14: Talked about how Mom-Mom locked them in a cabinet because they didn't clean up toys and was yelling at them, "Don't talk back."

March 15: At around 6:30 p.m. difficulty following directions; she was playing with Styrofoam even after she was asked to put it away. Hit Sister in the face with it, knocking her drink into her tooth and causing it to bleed. Got a time-out. After a couple of minutes of crying and telling mom, "You hurt my feelings," she said she wanted to apologize, ran to her sister to see her mouth, and apologized. Was able to move on.

*Woke up at 4:00 a.m. saying she had a Chuckee dream. Called out for potty, drink, and food. Did not fall back to sleep until after 5:30 a.m.

March 16: Good day: hyperactive and clingy at the dentist's.

March 17: OK day: upset after the psychiatrist visit because she wanted Chick fil A, poured water in the car purposefully in a compartment to try to get her way, and had conversation with Mom about actions and consequences; she understood and apologized. Passed a house in the city and she said it was Mom-Mom's. Talked about how that house had been haunted and Mom-Mom had given them a Chuckee doll. She then saw a dog and started talking about how Mom-Mom almost stole a dog and wanted them to help, but they didn't.

March 18: Good day.

March 19: Minor arguing at minigolf; took consequence and apologized to Sister.

March 20: Crying at night; told Dad she hated (Mom). She said her mom had a cage for her and her sister helped her mom trap her in a cage.

Week 6

March 21: Nurse called; she ate grass outside at recess. Overly hyperactive when visitors came. Good day overall. At times, talking like a baby. Has said she wants to be three.

March 22: Rough morning: woke up at 5:30 a.m. and asked for the light to be turned off. Twenty minutes later screaming out for light to be turned back on.

Babbling and crying about the grim reaper being real and giving her nightmares. Later, after Sister went to school, went in her room and was feeding the dog crayons. After therapy, fell asleep during the car ride. After lunch, refused to get out of the car to go to school. Took possibility of losing Easter basket to finally go in. At visit with Mom-Mom, she attempted to lock out the state worker to show Mom-Mom something (claimed she wanted to show a rash). Very hyperactive the rest of the night.

March 23: Increased tears throughout the day. First day of medication change. At the mall very active wanting to touch and see everything.

March 24: Good day: minor bouts of crying for little things (not wanting to eat the meat in her Lunchables, headphones not working, and so on).

March 25: OK day: difficulty with being out of routine for spring break and a lot of intermittent tears.

March 26: Great day: meltdown when she was hungry.

March 27: Very excited and hyperactive.

The Older One

Week 1

Over weekend: an invisible friend appeared; afraid to go into Friendly's because she had been there before and food got taken.

February 16: Rough evening. Lots of fighting with Sister; pouting and attention-seeking behavior such as whining, crying, and grabbing animals from her sister's calm-down area. Excessive need to make things a competition and want to win. Gave items to Sister and then took them back. Shared feelings about her real mom and discussed a closet hideout they had together filled with candy.

February 18: Attempted to use the phone to call other grandparent at the lice clinic. Frequent arguments with Sister, lying and attempting to escalate her sister in order to make herself the center of attention and/or appear helpful.

February 19: Attention-seeking behavior continued. Parents talked to her about being a big sister and what that meant.

February 20: Emotional manipulative behaviors observed: lying about her sister to get attention; when sharing that her sister was confined to a bathroom by her biological mom in the dark for a time-out, she defended her mom causing her sister to shut down. She then had a breakdown about not being able to see her mom's picture.

February 21: Received extra incentive points for being supportive of her sister, being well behaved at church and Applebee's, and cleaning up. Obsessed about seeing her mom's jail on the way to church. Continued lying about little things (when a movie came on, she said she met the actor; said she was in the movie, etc).

Both girls: obsessed with babies, love Chucky and other similar movies, and expressed difficulty with stepfather figure.

Week 2

February 22: Good day. Purposefully jumped in mud multiple times on the playground and then put mud on the slide. Working on having her showing respect and caring for things.

February 23: Difficulty picking out an outfit in the morning—kept wanting to wear summer dresses. After Sister wasn't feeling well, said her head hurt, stomach hurt, and she wished there was a delay and she didn't have to go to school. Went to the nurse at school multiple times until she called the foster mom. She insisted she was sick. At school, she was laughing and giggling in the office. No signs of illness. Later, she admitted she lied because she wanted to come home. In the tub she said how Grandpa died in a mermaid movie. When confronted with if she believed this was true, she said yes. When confronted further, she said no. Later in the tub, she said her sister threw a cup at her head. When the foster mom said no she didn't as she had watched the interaction, a weird smile spread over her face.

February 24: Very rough night: multiple temper tantrums, pouty, and screaming, "Go away; I don't want to talk to you," when she didn't like her present and wanted to switch with her sister even though it was the present she initially requested.

February 25: Up and down evening: continuation of pouty behavior; had to discuss disrespect, expressing feelings, and being honest.

February 26: Good day. Imaginary friend talk in the car along with discussion of being in a haunted house with her aunt where they ran out of the car, stole a wallet, and went to Dunkin' Donuts. At bowling lost ten points for pouty sulking during the game. Continuation of concern for her to be able to identify emotions and why she's feeling that way.

February 27: Very rough day. Locked the kitten and the dog in the cage telling them to fight in the basement. Did not understand why this was upsetting even though we had discussed proper treatment of animals and going in the basement without permission. No remorse evident and was able to shift back into happy mode even when the steak house arcade outing got taken away. When a former student in the fifth grade with autism came over to visit and play in the park, she battled for his attention; also almost hit her sister in the head with several branches while throwing them at the dog in the dog park. While watching Inside Out *and seeing foster parents cry at a scene, she mimicked the emotion to make herself cry. Her sister shared that she was faking. Continued fabrications of stories: her mom bought her a $100,000 car, but it crashed; her mom took her to see* Inside Out *in the theater; she said she hadn't gone to the bathroom for a bowel movement for four days (when confronted with this and the medical ramifications—she changed her story).*

February 28: Good day. A lot of talk about her mom on the way to church with grandiose stories; reinforced nice touches with animals and sharing. Did social stories and feeling apps at dinner, which she responded well to. When reminded there was a visit with Mom-Mom the next day at dinner, she shared she was upset because of what happened the last time she saw her; when prompted further she shared it was a story from when she was two. Her sister shared that last time their Mom-Mom almost broke her hip and died when she tripped on one of their toys, but they got her ice, and she was OK.

Week 3

February 29: The visit brought out a variety of behaviors for her. Once she was reminded of the visit and told the plan, her moods fluctuated from happy to pouty to sulking to zoning out. This was on the car ride over. During the visit serious regression occurred: weird attention seeking, demanding behavior, snatching items, yelling, running around, jumping on things, and purposefully locking her sister into a dark cabinet by grabbing a wooden chair and angling it on the door so her sister could not get out. This occurred at least two times within the foster parent's portion of observation behind the two-way mirror within a span of five minutes.

*On the ride home after the cabinet incident was addressed, Mom asked why both girls were not acting like themselves during the visit, referring to them being the polite, respectful, and caring girls toward one another that the foster parents usually observed. To this she responded that they wanted to act that way and their heads were telling them to but their bodies were not responding.

*Additionally both girls discussed how their stepmother had locked them in a room with pokes (nails) one time and also locked them out of the house once to which their dad came home to find them sitting on the front steps.

March 1:.Regression with playing and sharing with her sister. Throughout the evening we modeled appropriate turn-taking behavior having both girls reenact situations as needed when grabbing, snatching, and whining occurred. We continued to reinforce and model how to "use words" and "check in" during playtime. She kept interrupting adults and her sister while talking for everyone to focus on her. Was stopped and directed to wait her turn. Then when it was her turn was purposefully called on. Also a wand for her sister and a pencil for her were used as nonverbal cues to identify whose turn it was to speak during snack time as both girls were interrupting and talking excessively at the same time. While watching videos at bedtime with her as she asked, she flipped on the following: http://youtu. be/UK2fv9ACWCs.

We watched the first part with the cat in the well. I asked her, "What did this make you think? Did you feel anything during this video?" She couldn't think of anything and said she didn't feel anything while watching the video. We reviewed the theme of the video and how the boy learned from his mistake.

March 2: When she got home from school, she locked Dad behind the pet gate; said she was playing. Lost ten points and had a time-out. It was reinforced with her that "everyone has the right to feel safe in the house."

Talked to her and her sister. In the tub her sister shared that her mom, mom's boyfriend, and dad's girlfriend would lock them in places, including a cabinet that had a key lock. She shared that she in particular was locked in there for hours. The foster mom spoke to both girls saying that it was never OK to be locked anywhere like that, that she was sorry that happened, and that we could not lock *anyone or any animal anywhere like that. She shared to the older one that if she was thinking about those times to talk about it instead of "playing" by locking people and animals up. Lied about playing the Wii at school. When Mom shared she couldn't wait to see the Wii at her conference next week, she said it broke today. When asked if Mom should discuss it with her teacher, she said her teacher didn't want to talk about it. When asked what her teacher would say, she paused. When asked if there was really a Wii, she smiled, laughed, and said she was playing. They had a discussion about lying. Later looking at a photo album with Mom, she shared for every picture that she could do that, did that, or had been there. This happens all the time with new places or movies where she says she's met actors. She then shared that she wished she hadn't moved here because she missed her mom. She explained that even though she hadn't seen her mom in years, Mom-Mom showed her a picture on her phone the other day during the visit.*

Week 4

March 7: Difficulty following directions with Dad after school. On the way out the door as Dad said to get away from the door to not let the dog out, she pushed on the door, opened it, and the dog started to run out. Very well behaved at the restaurant. Lied about bringing Mom's phone in. Said she gave it to dad; then hid by the fridge. When it was found in the backseat, she still stuck to her story that she gave it to Dad on the way inside.

March 8: Elbowed Sister on purpose on the trampoline pushing her down; redirected and given verbal warning. While lying with Mom before bedtime, she talked about the different houses she's stayed in with family members: Dad and his girlfriend with her three-year-old child. She shared how they had to leave when the baby was born and stay with Mom-Mom for a couple days. Also shared that the little one went on the balcony in the middle of the night at Mom-Mom's because of sleepwalking.

March 9: OK day. Locked Ben (dog) out back and would not admit to it. Parents believe it happened when she said she was going down to get her backpack for homework time (overly concerned for Ben when Mom called for him indicating she knew something). Showed her sister scary pictures before bed.

March 10: Responding well to additional behavioral incentives.

March 11: Pouty behavior before visit: interesting reaction to life photo book (did not flip through the whole thing, and when she got to a page with her brother, she put her head down and cried). While playing at home, locked herself in the dog cage and said she was playing.

March 12: Rough day with sharing and following directions at Aaron's parents' house.

March 13: Pouting/sulking at the steak house when the focus and attention were not on her. Refused to admit to locking Ben out and had Kindle taken away for one week.

Week 5

March 14: Hit Sister in the mouth with the cheese can when attempting to snatch it: got time-out. Huge breakthrough after lying in Dad's arms weeping for twenty minutes—was able to talk about what she did. The foster parents modeled being honest, getting the consequence, and moving on. Later when doing charts, she was honest about locking Ben (dog) out the week before. When asked if she was trying to hurt him, she said no she just wanted him to get out his excess energy.

March 15: Got hit by Sister with Styrofoam and took it very well by accepting her sister's apology. Positive progress with sharing observed as well as positive sibling interaction.

March 16: Good day. Continued with positive behaviors. Minor poutiness.

March 17: Lied at the eye doctor's to try to get glasses.

March 18: Good day.

March 19: Minor arguing at minigolf; pouted at consequence of leaving but then got it together. At night talked about memories of Pop-Pop and holiday traditions.

March 20: Fantastic day. While lying down at night, she talked about how Mom's boyfriend tried to get her to lock her sister in a suitcase. Also talked about being left alone in the house with no adult; her sister and baby brother wandered outside, and other people found them and let them all stay with them. They had a six- or seven-year-old. Only stayed with them for a day. When back at home, Mom was asleep. Mom went into her boyfriend's brother's room to get her phone. There was a loud bang, and she saw Mom on the ground with blood pouring down her face. Said at night she sees bloody things; thinks dirty clothes are bloody.

Week 6

March 21: Great day! Some attention-seeking behavior with visitors but was easily redirected. Difficulty falling asleep. Fell asleep around 12:45 a.m.

March 22: Did a great job at the DSS visit and earned ten extra points.

March 23: Minor pouting at restaurant. Enjoyed troop meeting. Good night. Rough time falling asleep.

March 24: A lot of pouting and whining after school. Got upset when she tried to control the Easter egg hunt and boss her sister around. Lost the privilege of having the ice-cream cake when she couldn't eat it right away and whined excessively.

March 25: After she got the Easter candy eggs, she made a game where the little one could get an egg if she was good and then tried to control the ones she got. Faked crying and being upset as the parents and her sister were upset during the movie The Good Dinosaur. *Difficulty sleeping. When asked why, she said she had bad dreams and did not want to sleep. When asked further, she said she was worried about her baby brother and Mom being stabbed. When asked if she ever saw that, she said one time—a long time ago—in Kmart she saw a man stab the top of a car, and it really scared her. She said she pushed him, but Mom-Mom wouldn't remember because it was so long ago.*

March 26: Good day. Minor pouting at the steak house but got over it quickly.

March 27: Awesome day; got maximum incentive points.

March 26, 2016: Unsupervised visit with paternal grandparents. I text to tell the state worker the location and time prior to and after the visit. We are told by paternal grandparents that Mom-Mom has staked out our car and gotten our information. They are able to recite our address back to us and tell me when I bought my house and the amount I paid for it. Additionally, they shared that both girls have a trust fund in their names due to a lawsuit from their grandfather who passed away. They cannot access it until twenty-five, and the grandparents share that Mom-Mom and the biological mom hope to access it earlier, which is why they are fighting so hard for custody. All of this is shared with the state and our agency.

We were so freaked out by this. I get looking up people, as I do it all the time. I want to know whom I'm dealing with as well. However, we were promised by our agency that there would be anonymity. Now, we had to worry about drug addicts having our home address? I got into plenty of trouble when I was a teenager hanging out with a rough crowd of my own. There were many times that gangs of people showed up at my front door with intentions to fight. But I haven't been sixteen in a long time. The neighborhood fights and mace incidents were long behind me and were not things I wanted to have to contend with as an adult of thirty-five. The only way it made sense that she could have gotten our information was if she had staked out our car at one of these visits. We couldn't have a better time to get out of the state. Over the break, I would also have to make plans to get an additional security camera installed. Just great.

April 1, 2016: The state worker responds with the following e-mail. "Hello Chrissie, I am sorry to hear that your information was looked up by Mom-Mom. I do not know how Mom-Mom got your last name if you did not provide it to her. I have not provided any information to the girls' family members. It is likely possible that the paternal grand-parent gave Mom-Mom your last name. Unfortunately we cannot control what someone else does with public knowledge, or how they abuse their personal jobs in order to get private information. Also, with visits in the community with the paternal grandparents and you and Aaron staying with the girls during the visits, there should not be discussion about Mom-Mom, the bio parents, or the case in general in the presence of the girls."

This lazy bitch. *Seriously, that is your response? How about you give out your home address, then, and we will see how you feel? And yeah, the paternal grand-parents gave her our information and then told us about it. That makes no sense.* This was my internal thought pattern. I was losing all respect and patience for this worker, as it was becoming more and more evident that she was just in this as a job and not to actually care about the kids.

Our trip to Florida was a relaxing success. We had chunked the trip in steps for the little one to transition easier, and even though we had bought both girls three movies to watch on their devices on the plane, they were so excited that they chatted instead, each of them clinging to one of us throughout the entire ride. The night we arrived in Florida, it was very late. My mom's condo is amazingly beautiful and has a view of water out of each window. After we had gotten the girls acclimated, we said good night, only to walk by their room later and see both of them on their tiptoes looking out at the "Intracoastal Waterway" watching all the boats go by. It was clear they had never seen anything like that before and were in awe. It was definitely one of the precious moments that made the hell of combating with the visits and system worthwhile. On the first day at the beach, when the little one's toes touched the sand, her face lit up. She was such a sensory child and could not believe the sensation her feet sinking in the sand. For each step she was mesmerized, only becoming more engrossed when she saw the all-powerful ocean. We spent almost the entire trip in the water, either at the beach or by the pool. It was the first time with both girls that we had consistently calm and peaceful days. Their demeanor had changed, and you would never know that they weren't just "normal" girls on vacation with their family. Of course, we also spoiled them rotten, buying toy after toy and anything else their hearts desired. It was a wonderful trip for us as a family. I only wished we could keep that content and happy feeling with us always.

When spring break was over, it was time for me to return to work. Since the little one thrived so much with an adult home in the morning, we had decided that Aaron would resign from his position to stay home with her and take her to her appointments. I loved the girls, but being a stay-at-home mom was not for me. I thrived the most in my job environment. Not that being a stay-at-home mom isn't a job, because dear God, it was the most difficult one I had ever had to do. The constant mess even though you had spent most of the day cleaning up, the endless pile of growing laundry, pieces of things, just things everywhere, and oh dear, the constant soggy state of the bathroom rugs. No matter what bath mat I got or how many towels I had, the bathroom floor might as well have been its own body of water. Not to mention the endless battle with food, homework, and bedtime. I was ready for adult conversation. Yes, I would be dealing with kids, but I knew none of their temper tantrums would even compare to those of my little one. She had prepped me well while I was off, so I was ready to be the best behavioral interventionist I could be, equipped with all the calm-down resources she no longer used.

It was so great to be back at work in a routine I knew and surrounded by people who loved me. Also, being able to talk with other adults was amazing. As I was finishing up a great first day back, sitting in a meeting with my principal and a teacher, I saw an e-mail come across from the state worker. She was requesting a date for a visit with the girls' biological mom. What? And it was to be for later this week? My stomach flipped. I felt sick. I excused myself and called Aaron. We were both in shock. Hadn't they just told us last month that it would be a while?

April 4, 2016: We are notified via e-mail that the state worker is setting up a visit for the girls with their biological mom, and it can either occur on April 7, April 11, or April 12. When we asked for clarification of this visit and expectations, we never received a return phone call. When we asked via e-mail for clarification, we never received a response.

With no response from the state worker on why this was occurring so fast, Aaron, who had taken the reins on communication since I was back at work, sent the e-mail below.

April 5, 2016: E-mail from us: "Hi everyone, I have tried calling everyone in an effort to understand why it is that the visit with biological mom and her daughters (that are under our care) is happening so soon. As we understood the situation, this type of visit was not supposed to happen for a while. We also expected more notice for such an event as to give ample time for the girls to mentally prepare for such an occasion. It was also recommended by the little one's therapist that this not happen for a while because of the trauma that she endured under the watch of her biological mother. We are therefore, confused as to why it is that the powers that be think this is a good idea. If we could get some clarification in regards to why this meeting is happening so rapidly we would be able to feel more at ease. To be frank, at this juncture, we feel as though this meeting would have a negative impact on the girls' mental state. If you wouldn't mind getting back to me and my wife before the reunion takes place, we would be very grateful." We never get a response.

Really, not even a phone call, text, or anything. It looked like this was happening, so we might as well get it over with. And we had to meet her. I was an emotional wreck. I have known and loved many drug addicts in my lifetime, specifically friends who had been addicted to heroin. Hell, I had even lost one of them when I was sixteen to a suicide as a result of withdrawal from heroin. I was the one who advocated for parents in this woman's situation within my school, assisting them in any way I could. Why was this so hard? I guess because I also loved these girls as if they were my own, and just knowing she could beat, confine, and bully the little one disgusted me. And I had no idea how she was going to react. I had been warned about her volatile hostility, which displayed itself pretty much all the time. But maybe that was just all a result of her addiction. Maybe when I met her and she met me, we could come to a consensus about these two girls we both loved in our own way in regard to them having happy, healthy lives.

I was terrified. So I did what I always do when I'm full of fear—have a lot of people pray for me and wear a really awesome, kick-ass outfit. I chose my half-leather, somewhat tight but stylish black dress with boots. It stated "professional," but also "don't fuck with me." Just the message I wanted to send. I called in all reinforcements to say a prayer for me during this meeting. I was really going to need to be a Christian for this. I didn't know if I could do it. Not to mention, we also had to prep the girls for the meeting. They hadn't seen their biological mother in over a year, and so they were a ball of mixed emotions, displaying them in different ways.

The day went fast, thanks to work meetings, and it wasn't long before I was racing out of the office early. I had never left early or been absent so much since getting the girls. I saw and understood now how work takes a backseat to your children. I stopped home and picked up Aaron and the girls, and we were on our way, not quite sure what to expect. As we were getting out of the car, I saw a woman and a baby carriage in the distance. I had looked up pictures of their biological mom, but this did not appear to resemble the woman I had seen. She looked rough, haggard, and appeared to be panhandling, using the baby in the carriage to get people to feel sympathetic and give her money. No, that couldn't be her. Soon we were ushered back into the same room where our little one had been locked in the cabinet. The girls were taken with another worker, and we awaited the arrival of Bio-Mom. The room was crowded with the state worker, our worker, Aaron, and me. The supervisor was watching behind the two-way mirror. I had no idea what to expect. I didn't know if this woman was going to hit me, cuss me out, or what. I just knew, in spite of everything, I had to maintain my composure and be the bigger person, for the girls, no matter what came my way.

When she walked in, I was startled to see that it was in fact the mother I had seen in the parking lot. The pictures I had looked up must have been super outdated. I went over to greet her, handing her a picture of the girls with the Easter bunny. As she attempted to shake my hand, she refused to look me in the eye, and her arm hung limp like a wet noodle, indicating that she was going to make little effort to connect with me. Her first words were, "The girls will be coming home with me."

Well, hello to you too!

She continued going on and on about her program and then demanding that she have overnight visits with the girls at her halfway house. *Are you serious? First of all, why would you want them in that environment? Second, is anyone in this room going to set this woman straight?* I looked to the workers. As always, they remained silent. Not me though. I politely explained that the little one had PTSD and what that entailed. She blew me off, stating that she had that. In my best special-education explanation that I would convey to any parent, I continued. Nope, she blew me off, indicating that she didn't believe in diagnoses, because after everything she kept saying "I had that." I wanted to say, yes, you had that, and we are sitting here because you were a drug addict who abused your children and got sent to jail. That is not exactly a well-adjusted person and is not something I would think a mother would want for her daughter.

As we went through the activities of the girls and their accomplishments with us over the past couple of months, she either scoffed or just plain ignored us, talking instead directly to the state worker about herself. Throughout the whole time, she was mechanically manhandling the one-month-old. There appeared to be little to no emotion there. When the worker shared that the little one would have to have dental surgery because of two rotting teeth—you know, because she had never taken them to the dentist—she rolled her eyes. Wow, really? I hung in there though, going along with the tone of the room—being diplomatic and stating that we were just taking care of her girls until she could, commending her on creating such wonderful children, and asking her if she had any questions about us, adding that I would want to know more about the people taking care of my children. Nope, no questions for us. She refused to look us in the eye and dismissed almost everything that came out of my mouth. Not to mention that she was talking about overnight visits as if they were going to happen the next day. Was there something I didn't know? I had no trust in these workers at this point.

April 7, 2016: Visit occurred with the biological mom, state worker, state supervisor observing, our agency worker, and us (foster parents). We had an icebreaker in which the biological mom shared that her children would be coming home with her. She dismissed the little one's diagnosis of PTSD and stated how she wanted the girls to have overnight visitation with her at her program as soon as possible. We were as professional as possible, asking her if she had any questions for us and telling her that we were only taking care of her kids until she could. We reiterated that we understood the goal was reunification. We also gave her an Easter picture of the girls. After twenty minutes of our icebreaker, the girls were brought in to visit with her and the newborn baby. We met with both our worker and the state worker in the hallway. The state worker said that she'd never had an initial meeting go so well. The supervisor walked by and asked how we were doing. We asked about the recommendations from the therapist, and the state worker stated she never received it. I reminded her about our meeting in February where the recommendation was given for the little one to have a slow transition to visits with Mom. She said she never received it in writing. I shared that the therapist's office had called me requesting the state's information weeks prior, so I knew it had been sent.

Our agency worker walked us out to the parking lot. She stated, "I couldn't say it in there, because I didn't know who was listening, but you have to be careful what you say, or 'they' could take the girls away. Especially if you advocate too much!" What the hell did that mean? Where was I, in prison, on *Big Brother*? Was I Jason Bourne, and I didn't know it? Basically, shut my mouth, play by the rules, and take the check. Um, while I watched little girls I loved like my daughters deteriorate. That is not even within my capacity to do. I listened respectfully, processing the intended "read between the lines" message, thanked her for being there even though she remained silent throughout the interaction, and retreated to the car, not having any idea what to expect. It felt like at any minute the girls could be carted off and possibly be staying for overnight visits at a halfway house.

We were called thirty minutes early to come get the girls, as the little one was displaying significant regression, and their biological mother had to be debriefed. We were told that visits with the biological mom would be weekly. I was sickened. They were going to make us endure this every week.

April 7 to May 26: Visitation with the biological mom has an impact on the little one. Regression and concerns are documented and shared with the state. Concerns were shared in regard to the biological mom slipping her phone number to the girls along with notes while in the supervised visits. Additionally, she gave them photos of her boyfriend in a "Family" album. The little one displays concerning sexualized behavior such as licking the private parts of stuffed animals, attempting to pose for naked selfies, kissing boys, and sitting in boys' laps on the bus. At one meltdown at school where foster parents were called to come intervene, she was under a cafeteria table refusing to get up, yelling her mom's name, and repeatedly saying she was mean. When the foster mom got to the school, the little one was with the principal in the office. She repeated over and over again that she needed to have a boyfriend. The little one demonstrated domestic violence with dolls after a visit with the biological mom. We were told by the state that visits were going "very well." Within the visits we had, three ended early, and the biological mother was not able to attend due to starting a fight at her program and being on lockdown "reflection time."

April 12, 2016: E-mail from the therapist to the state worker and the girls' attorney: "We spoke a few weeks ago. Recent and planned visits with the little one's biological mother cause me significant concern about her well-being. Her symptoms are extremely activated as a result of the visit last Thursday and continue to escalate in anticipation of the visit scheduled for this Thursday. I would like to inform you of specifics and my recommendations. You can access this written information in her medical record which the state and/or you can access through our medical records department. Also, please feel free to call me to discuss the case."

April 21, 2016: Dentist communication. The state worker had been previously informed on April 5, 2016, via e-mail that she or a DSS worker needed to be in attendance for the little one's dental hospitalization. The dentist had shared that her office had tried to call and left a message the week before but had not heard back. The date was chosen on the basis of her availability. The day prior to the scheduled surgery, the dentist tried to speak with her. The dentist had again left a message stating she would not be able to attend. They shared that they were unable to reach her and that if a worker was not in attendance, the surgery could not proceed. After our e-mail, she called back to inform us that another worker would be in attendance; however, she did not have her number.

I had worked out a day off and scheduled my whole life around this damn dental-surgery date, and I was a nervous wreck for my little one. Having just had surgery the year before, I knew the process she was in for with getting paperwork, not eating, and having to wait. Now they were telling me it may have to be rescheduled due to what I perceived as the state worker's damn incompetence. So she was sending a sub. Great, but we didn't know her name, number, or anything. Just what I like to be, unprepared. The state worker did not seem at all concerned with the hell my little one was going to have to endure for this surgery. She was five, had ADHD, had never seen a dentist, would be going under anesthesia, and had to have two rotting teeth extracted along with baby root canals. Was my agency there? Nope, not at all. It was Aaron and I being Mommy and Daddy, holding her hand, ensuring everything would be OK, and telling her that when it was all done, she could get her snow-cone reward. I was so anxious and worried for her.

After the debacle with the substitute state worker, we were finally taken back, where she had to wait for what seemed like forever. The hospital staff were amazing. Seeing our paperwork and our interaction with the little one, they were very empathetic and kind to our plight. They saw how much we loved her. In turn, they were also quite disgusted with the late state worker, indicating that their experiences with situations like this before had been even more unpleasant. At one point, the little one could no longer control the ADHD and leaped off the bed. We were sure she was making a run for it. Thankfully, Aaron was there to catch her. My iPhone and her Kindle could only sustain her attention for so long. When the anesthesiologist came along and said the medicine he was going to give her tasted like bubble gum, I almost admired her for her natural, no-bullshit reaction of taking one sip and dribbling the rest out of her mouth onto her gown. She was not a child you could bullshit by any means. God, I loved her feisty little self!

When a ninety-year-old woman was wheeled into the curtain close to us, wailing and screaming, she settled down, trying to make sense of the whole experience. Finally, she was wheeled off to surgery at 2:30 p.m. She hadn't eaten since ten o'clock the night before. Poor baby! I prayed she would be strong and OK. I was a hot mess of worry. Aaron left because he had to pick up the older one from the bus stop, and then they would both return. Surprise, surprise, no text from the state worker. She obviously cared a whole lot about the little one's well-being. Our agency had e-mailed me on a separate issue, so I took the time in the waiting room to call them back. The supervisor shared she was glad the procedure was able to take place with the difficulty that had occurred. *Yeah, no thanks to your involvement.*

The dentist came out shortly after my phone call, and I was immediately relieved on hearing that the procedure went very well. Knowing how much I loved this little girl, she said that she would pray for our case but that, no matter what, I had given her a gift by having this procedure done, as she had to be in a lot of pain due to the state of her mouth. When I saw her, OK and healthy, lying on the bed, eyes lighting up when she saw me, my heart filled with joy. My little rock star! She was so tough. Immediately, she stated how hungry she was, and I couldn't blame her. Before the nurse had even come to us with juice and a snack, she had gone through two packages of fruit snacks from the arsenal in my purse. Every mom needs an arsenal. It is an unwritten rule. To the nurse's amazement, she downed two packages of goldfish, two juices, and one cookie and took several for the road with no indication that she had any pain at all when chewing. She was such a tough little girl. We met Aaron and her sister right outside of the hospital, with her new fish pillow in tow as a reward for making it through the surgery from the hospital staff. Of course, I had promised her two snowballs, and that was all she wanted, so off we went. I couldn't believe how fast she was recovering. I had expected her to be out of it all night, but nope, she was happy and healthy and appeared to be relieved. I wondered just how much pain her mouth had been causing her, and she just hadn't said anything.

April 22, 2016: The substitute state worker was late, signed one thing, and left. We had to get her to come back to finish the registration process in order for the little one's procedure to occur.

Two days after the dental procedure, I became sicker than I had been in quite some time. In fact, not since seven years earlier when I had become an assistant principal had I been so sick. I had a 103-degree temperature and did not have the strength to get out of bed, but as a mom, you know you do not get sick days. Both girls crawled in bed with me, and we had TV marathons. I didn't want to infect them, but they refused to leave my side. I had to call out of work, but of course the day after was a day off for the girls, so they were home. At that point, I had passed my germs on to Aaron, so we were both struggling with this flu/cold/plague situation, trying to maintain some composure as parents. There is certainly no manual for this in training. It wasn't long before both girls were sick as well. Of course we had a visit scheduled for that day with Mom-Mom, so I had to reach out to the state worker. She took her sweet time responding, asking if both girls were out of school. Really, you don't know they have the day off? Wow, you are competent at your job. I texted her back to tell her that there was no school, to which I got back, "Well, if they're sick, then we will reschedule." That only took seven hours. Thank you so much. It was so frustrating to have to adhere to someone else to make decisions for little people whom you considered to be your children.

Two days later, I was getting worse. The little one was fully recovered. I assumed that perhaps the antibiotics she was on from her procedure had knocked it out of her but am not a medical doctor. The older one had my fever temperature as well. She stayed home from school, and I again had to tell the worker she wouldn't be able to make the visit. The worker then asked if she had been to the doctor yet. Aaron took the reins on the response, stating that she had gotten better and then deteriorated, and if it persisted, we would go to the doctor. I wondered how their biological mother would feel about only having the little one for the visit that day, as she clearly favored the older one. I also was concerned about what she would do to the little one. The older one didn't seem fazed or upset to miss a visit, stating, "I'm happy I get to spend time with my mommy." Mommy—me, that was. So she and I snuggled up watching TV and being sick, while Aaron and the little one headed off to the dreaded visit. We had a grand time together. When they returned, Aaron looked depleted and exasperated. The little one bounded in proclaiming that "Mommy was rich now," thanks to her boyfriend, and he was no longer going to be mean. He was going to treat them like little flowers. Clearly, another very appropriate conversation had occurred with their visit. When asked about how their mom felt about the older one not being there, the little one conveyed she had looked ready to cry. The older one pretty much ignored all that came out of the little one's mouth about their mom and the visit. She was too engrossed in continuing to stake her claim on her time with me. It was a very weird dynamic between the two of them.

So at the beginning of May, I had rather had enough. I felt like a shell of a human being having to watch the mental anguish the girls were going through as a result of the visits, especially my little one. Her dissociation had escalated full on into different personalities, and her violent outbursts were increasing, along with her sexualized behavior and night terrors that horrified me. Our agency acted as though they were supporting us while collaborating with the state. But the result was that no one was doing anything to assist the girls. It wasn't even in the damn court order that they had to have visitation with their mother. But it didn't matter, because reunification was always the plan, until there was enough evidence to prove that it shouldn't be, and I just needed to hang in there until the following October. I was at my wits' end, so I decided to take it up a notch. I had contacts within my school community for the senator who was my school's former PTA president years before I got there, as well as a councilman who rightfully considered himself a part of our community, so I penned the following impassioned plea:

Good Morning Senator and Councilman,

I'm reaching out to you this morning as a fellow community member and an advocate of children in hopes that you will be able to direct me to someone I can speak to about the deplorable condition of the Department of Social Services Foster Care System. As an assistant principal for the past seven years who has been the IEP chair in an educational system, there is nothing that I will not do to advocate for a child. We have so many policies and procedures that are designed to help kids get what they need and although our system is not perfect, we are constantly looking for ways to make it better in order to serve the community it is supposed to protect. I think that is why I have been so shocked being on the other side of things with Social Services working with my agency to attempt to foster to adopt two little girls who have been in the system for years. Instead of the caseworker and supervisor advocating for the best interests of my girls, instead, they advocate for the constitutional rights of the biological parent stating that it is the system and they are just checking off a list of things given down from people above and to which they have no control over. With my personal case, my little one's therapist has recommended no more visits with her biological mom as it will continue re-traumatize her due to her PTSD from the documented abuse. However, the attorney and the system all refuse to follow that recommendation due to the way the system works. Their mother is in a court appointed program out of prison that instead of focusing on the case at hand is just trying to push her through to be a success story. That is what we have been told by the attorney involved as we attempted to advocate for our kids. Then, we have been told that if we advocate too much, the state will take them out of our care and give them to a family who is not as much "trouble" in spite of what is in the best interest of the kids because they do not want to be bothered. They are confused as to why we are not just focused on "housing" these little girls like we are supposed to. We love them very much but as we have been told, have no voice in their case. Additionally, as the state worker shared, there is currently a case in the system where the biological parent hears voices and is threatening to kill their kids where the goal continues to be reunification. In another case, a biological parent was convicted of murder, got their kids back and now they are once again in foster care. My husband and I are going to continue to fight this losing battle in an attempt to keep our girls although we know they are slated to go back to their mom who will continue to sell their food stamps and use them for state money. However, we would like to talk to lawmakers or anyone that could possibly make a difference in changing this system for the better so it protects the children it claims to in its title: Child Protective Services. Right now, there are so many kids suffering due to the antiquated design of the system in MD and no one is stepping up to try to change anything which is why I had to reach out to you. This is wasting so much state money with people who are taking advantage of this current system in place. Anyone you could direct me to would be so greatly appreciated. Thank you so much for your time and for all you do.

May 4, 2016: E-mail from the state worker: "Hello, I just wanted to let you all know that we are arranging the FTDM for Monday at 11:00 a.m. In addition to the FTDM, I have arranged for a forensic interview to take place for the girls at 11:00 a.m. A social worker from our sex abuse unit will interview the girls. This will take place at the Child Advocacy Center that is located on the side of our building. (This is the door you all went through when we had our initial icebreaker with the paternal grandparents.) Additionally, our FTDMs are usually about 2 hours. We will have child care services for the girls after the interview while we are in the meeting. Someone from our FTDM unit will contact you all with the details of the meeting but I just wanted to give you a heads up. If you have any questions let me know." We did follow up and called the state worker with questions that evening. We never heard from a facilitator and received a text from the state worker on May 5, 2016, asking us to be at the forensic interview ten minutes early. I texted back stating our agency worker had tried to reach her and asked if she had heard back. I did not receive a response until Monday morning when I was on my way to the meeting.

—⎯⎯⎯⎯⎯

An e-mail came from our social worker in the middle of the week. It was actually rather alienating, given the insider language that was used. It read something like, "We have an FTDM meeting coming up, and all parties will be there." I remember looking at that e-mail and wondering just what in the hell an FTDM was. Chrissie called me shortly after the e-mail came in and sounded unhappy.

"What is an FTDM?" she asked, sounding a little more than frustrated. I absolutely understood where she was coming from. None of this process had worked out the way that we had expected, and it was starting to give us both a bitter taste in our mouths for the Department of Social Services and even our adoption facility.

"I have no idea what that is," I replied, wondering why our social worker would use an acronym like that with a couple that was new to the system. That nomenclature isn't in a damn handbook.

"I'll google it and figure it out," I said, in an effort to take some of the anxiety off Chrissie's mind. We said our good-byes and hung up to continue our respective days.

I took to Google and punched the letters FTDM into the search bar. The results didn't yield anything immediately, but about five hits down, there was something that sounded reasonably close to the situation we were handling. FTDM: family team decision-making meeting.

Wow, Department of Social Services. Just—wow. I rubbed my face with my hands, knowing that this was not going to be an enjoyable or pleasant engagement. We had already met Bio-Mom, and she was a complete lunatic in the smallest of closed-door settings. What was going to happen when she was surrounded by the Department of Social Services people, our agency workers, and possibly lawyers from all sides? Jesus, this was going to be a nightmare. The meeting was to be held three days after the e-mail was sent, and boy, if that day didn't come zooming up to us like it was the goddamned Flash.

_____

We were headed out of town that weekend to take the girls to Aaron's family's house in Deep Creek in order to celebrate my first Mother's Day. That e-mail rattled me and shook me to my core. First of all, what the hell was an FTDM? I finally understood what it felt like to be a parent at my team meetings with all the acronyms. I got a text from Aaron that it meant "family team decision-making meeting." What did that entail? Who would be there? Would they take the girls from us that day? I had no idea; I just knew that all

I felt was panic and fear. Then, I realized what they would have to endure in a forensic interview. I didn't think they were going to open up to a complete stranger. Hell, it had taken them months to open up about certain abuse with us. This just continued to get harder. And yet, I had to maintain. I had to be "Mommy." So that is what I did, and we gave them the most fun weekend we could in Deep Creek, staying in a gorgeous, large house that they loved, going to the arcades, splashing through the lake, go-kart racing, and spoiling them rotten with whatever they wanted. In the midst of the cloud of unsettling uncertainty, it was a nice getaway.

> May 6, 2016: The little one has a night terror where she recounts "Mom's boyfriend" stealing her, locking her in a box, and taping her mouth shut. She shares that he touched her in the private area. This is e-mailed to the state worker in preparation for the interview.

This was enough, right? Surely they would be able to act on this accusation. I had showed them the pictures of the boyfriend's social-media page, his cover page laced with a vial of cocaine, hundred-dollar bills, and pot leaves. This was the house the girls would be going back to. All I heard from the state worker was that he was not a party to the case and that the house and everyone occupying it would have to pass a home inspection. I later heard from people who passed the home inspection that it was a joke and not nearly as extensive as the one we had to go through with our private agency.

—⌒—

We drove to the Department of Social Services building with the girls in tow, feeling like we would rather be sitting on the surface of the sun than be at that fucking building.

Upon entering we found that, surprise! No one was ready for us yet. *Huh! That's weird! Oh well, I guess three days isn't enough to plan a giant fuck-off meeting with fifteen people involved. Oh! Some of you are late, and you don't have the room ready for us to meet in? No worries! We will just wait out here in the lobby. We will go ahead and do that with Bio-Mom sitting directly across from us.*

It was a horrific twenty-minute wait with the girls bouncing back and forth between their biological mother and Chrissie. I thought that my wife was going to lose it right there in the waiting room and just start beating the hell out of the twenty-five-year-old fuckup that was the girls' mom.

An employee finally stuck her head into the oven that had once been the lobby and let us know that a room had finally been emptied and readied for our "meeting." We walked through the cubicles of the lovely offices of the Department of Social Services. It felt like a maze of despair. Each twist and turn made me feel more depressed than the last. The conference room that we were to be spending the next couple of hours in was finally in sight, and I wanted to ram my fist into a wall.

—6

May 7, 2016: At the Sex Abuse Center, they have no record of us coming for an interview. There is no state worker there to greet us. We have to call the state worker several times to get her on the phone. She is not aware of the name of the person who will be interviewing us. She rolls her eyes, clearly indicating her disgust with the state worker. Once the girls are interviewed, the interviewer speaks with me. She had no record of the most recent account, so I shared it with her.

In the waiting area for the FTDM meeting, we walked over and saw Mom-Mom. Then the biological mom and baby walked into the waiting area, followed by our agency's worker and supervisor. No state worker was present or facilitating interactions in the waiting area. The biological mom was on the phone with her boyfriend, who was on his way to come take care of her baby while she attended the meeting. There was no childcare set up. The state workers arrived and perceivably scrambled around to find available workers to watch the children. The concern that they could run into their "alleged abuser" was shared by us and our agency worker to try to get the children out of the waiting area and into childcare.

During the meeting, the biological mom cursed, "Fuck the ground rules! I don't give a fuck about her fucking ground rules," and walked out of the meeting after the psychiatrist and therapist shared on the phone that they had recommended and still recommended for visits with the biological mom for the little one to stop because of her fragile mental state. As a result of the biological mother's conduct in the meeting and frequent interjections on topics about herself that did not have to do with the little one, the meeting was over three hours long. The rest of the FTDM was that all participants (paternal grandparents, Mom-Mom, state workers, agency workers, and us, the foster parents) agreed that the little one should start with the outpatient program. When the biological mom came back into the meeting, she also agreed. The supervisor did sneak us out with the girls through the back door so that we did not run into the alleged abuser boyfriend. It was also recommended that the little one have play therapy at the Sex Abuse Center, since the forensic interview was inconclusive but concerning.

⤶

This just needs to be done and over with. My brain kept screaming, *Done!* But sadly, no, this actually had to happen. The total roster for this meeting read like a modern superhero movie. There was Chrissie and me, three of our agency's workers (who would go on to say literally nothing throughout the meeting), Bio-Mom and her lovely mother, the lovely paternal grandparents (that term was not sarcastic—we actually are very fond of them), a supervisor from the Department of Social Services, the girls' caseworker (she is an awful human being), and the mediator. And that was not all! On the phone we had the girls' psychiatrist, court-appointed counselor, school counselor, and schoolteacher!

I remember feeling very angry as I looked across the mammoth wood-stained table at the girls' biological mother. She was a twenty-five-year-old girl. She had four children already, and two of them were in our custody because she was too much of a fuckup to be trusted with their lives. And there she was, right across the table, sitting on her knees in a swivel chair like she was a twelve-year-old at a family dinner.

Can you not comport yourself like a goddamned adult for five minutes, you [you can imagine what words I was using to fill in the blank]? It's best I don't write out the rest of my thoughts there. It might be a little much, and I don't like to judge. Needless to say, Bio-Mom was a trap wreck of a human being. On multiple occasions she got up and paced around the room, acting like she was surrounded by crazy people, when the only crazy person I saw was her. She would throw fits every time we mentioned the illnesses the little one suffered from—ADHD, PTSD, and other forms of specific disorders resulting from neglect and abuse. Every single time we mentioned a problem, Bio-Mom chimed in, "I had that! I do that!" and "So do I!" Every single time, she let it be known that every aberrant behavior that the little one presented, she had done the same as a child. This drove us mad.

PTSD is not an inherited mental aberration, you fucking moron! I remember thinking. In regard to the little one's self-harm: "I mean, I did that too! Y'all are fuckin crazy!" This chick was absolutely out of her mind. And the state wanted these two little beautiful girls back in her care.

"How much longer are we going to have to endure this?" Chrissie asked one of our workers. In true form, they both shrugged and gave us noncommittal facial expressions. The facilitator then turned on Chrissie and said that the biological mother had a right to her feelings. The meeting went on and on. Toward the end, the trauma therapist and the psychiatrist stated, in no uncertain terms, that Bio-Mom was causing an undue amount of psychological harm to the little one. At that she stormed out of the room, despite the protest of her mother. From there, we had some real discussion. But Bio-Mom returned, and in no less crazy a state of mind. Soon we learned that Bio-Mom had summoned the dreaded drug-dealer boyfriend. He was to be Bio-Mom's means of transportation from the meeting. This guy, who had caused all manner of havoc in the girls' lives, was to be in the building that housed people meant to protect them.

The meeting came to a close, and Chrissie and I were ushered out of the conference room hurriedly and quietly. We were quickly transported to the area where the girls had stayed during the meeting and escorted out through what was essentially the back door. This was all for the purpose of avoiding the dreaded drug-dealer boyfriend. I couldn't believe this was happening. It felt like a scene out of a Jason Bourne movie.

I hate this, I remember thinking to myself. *And this is what these people want for the girls?* I felt the veins in my head pulse with rage. *What is wrong with these people?*

⟶ᴐ

I have been a party to many meetings and conferences within the thirteen years I have been in education. A lot of them have been unique. Some of them have been hostile. Never have I been in one that was this volatile, unprofessional, and lengthy. I had a very difficult time not jumping in to facilitate. I wanted to leave so many times, as we took the brunt of all her hostility, all her anger. She took no responsibility for the fact that we were all gathered around the table because of her actions. Instead, she stated that they should go back with the grandmother, that she didn't know why they called us Mommy and Daddy (implying we forced them to), and that we weren't family and would never see them again. She went on and on about herself: how she'd had that each time a disability was discussed, and she didn't know where the sexualized behavior would come from, because she was a "prude." Right, that's why she had four kids at the age of twenty-five. I just cringed on the inside. She kept saying how she thought that overnight visits or more contact with her would be what the little one needed, because, you know, she was the mom. I wanted to slap her across the face to come to her senses. She was the damn reason the little one was displaying all these symptoms.

She stated how she could slip a cell phone to the little one during a visit so they could call her. I was flabbergasted at the facilitator in the room allowing her to continue, let alone write some of her far-fetched ideas on the whiteboard as possible solutions. Somehow, I remained very calm on my exterior, attempting to placate her by saying that we didn't know what was causing the little one to react like this, but perhaps, as a result of some things she saw or experienced, the mother was triggering it. The grandparents confirmed this. God, I was thankful they were there. The paternal grandmother seemed to be at least someone the biological mother listened to and respected.

During the meeting, Mom-Mom had outright asked us our intentions. As honest and straightforward as I am, I leveled with her that we were a pre-adoptive resource. When we were presented with this case, we thought it was a case for adoption. By the time we found out differently, we already loved the girls. We understood the plan now and just wanted what was best for them. I saw her calm down, and throughout this meeting for the first time, she and I seemed to come to a nonverbal mutual level of respect. The tables had turned in our rapport, and I could sense she at least trusted what I was saying in the best interest of the little one. I knew she was misguided, but I also knew she loved those girls deeply in her own way. I probably gained the most respect for her when she turned to our agency's worker and supervisor, pointing and twirling her finger around, accusingly asking them, "And what do you do?" Because as always, they had remained silent, like they were statues just placed in seats in the room. Even Aaron and I turned our eyes to them, because to date we couldn't figure out their damn role except as one more entity we had to communicate our every movement with.

For three and a half hours, we sat in this damn meeting, going around and around with the biological mom's psychobabble about herself. We listened to the little one's teacher and guidance counselor. They shared experiences that illustrated the positive rapport the little one had with us and the follow-up interventions we had done as a result of behavioral concerns. The teacher was very clear that the little one always asked for her "assistant-principal mommy." This made the biological mom scoff and roll her eyes. While on the phone with the therapist, the state worker spoke up, saying, "I have a concern." She said this two more times and then proceeded to ask about things that were occurring in our care, such as "baby time" (ten minutes of baby time the therapist had recommended we give the little one each day as a result of her internal need to be a baby). If I could have gone across the table and dragged this worker by her weave, I would have. What the fuck? She couldn't have addressed these concerns with us prior to having everyone in the room? Jesus, the family already hated us enough. I would professionally cuss her out later.

Her little exploits about her concerns didn't matter, though, as we continued to receive praise for all that we were doing from the trauma therapist and psychiatrist. They both articulated that, because of the little one's deteriorating mental state, visits should be stopped. At that point, the mother hurled expletives and left the room. I looked around the table. The state worker went chasing after her like a little puppy dog. The grandparents, Aaron, and I all looked somewhat relieved. Now, we could finally get somewhere. The state worker came back twenty minutes later with a defeated look on her face, mumbling that the mother might come back or not. I would rather she didn't. After this performance, how in the hell could all these people think she was capable of raising her children? She couldn't even control herself for more than five minutes in a professional meeting. I was baffled that this was the situation I was in.

To my discomfort, the mother did end up coming back after Mom-Mom called her. The supervisor then took it upon herself to say how worried she was about us because we had gone into this hoping for adoption, and she didn't want to prevent us from continuing on with adopting other kids. Again, really appropriate to do this in such an open forum. I had hit my limit. *You want to air this shit out in this open forum? Get ready for me to professionally level you.* Which was exactly what I did by taking a beat and saying, "This experience has made us realize that we are done with fostering to adopt, so we would not want to take another case. And yes, we had wanted to adopt; however, we fell in love with these girls and want to help them. We could not bear it if they went to another foster home, because in the one they were placed in the weekend when they were in foster care in the fall, they were beaten." To that, everyone took a collective deep breath indicating their exasperation, like they couldn't believe that had occurred. The biological mom turned to the paternal grandmother, who confirmed my account, adding that the woman in that home overmedicated the little one because there were six other kids running around, and she didn't know what to do with her. Again, this meeting made me feel like we were the criminals because of the way the state treated us, and again, our agency stood by silently allowing it to happen. Our every move was being questioned, and now our emotional and mental state was being called into question. God, I just wanted to tell them all to fuck off. But this was not about me. It was about my baby, and I would do whatever I needed to, even if it meant swallowing my humility.

Somehow the meeting ended with all of us coming to a consensus that the little one needed the outpatient program immediately. That was my goal coming in, so no matter how much I had emotionally been beaten and abused by her mother and the state, it was worth it for her to get what she needed. They also felt like she would need additional play therapy, since the results of the forensic interview were inconclusive. When Aaron stated that she received play therapy at the trauma center, the supervisor dismissed that, stating that they would set up additional therapy on the side where we had met at the appointment that morning. Even though it would be yet another appointment, it would be in her best interest and could possibly lead to that boyfriend being charged, so it was worth it. Since the boyfriend was still in the lobby, the supervisor sneaked us around the maze of offices and out the back into the rain. What a horrible, mentally depleting experience! The girls looked like playing with the social worker had not fazed them, but because they were there so long with no school or lunch, we all agreed we needed to head to the steak house with their favorite arcade. Of course, it wasn't twenty minutes before I got a call from our agency's supervisor. She just wanted to check in, blah, blah, blah. I wanted to ask what the hell her job was, because they had not advocated or stood up for us at all.

> May 11, 2016: E-mail from us to the state worker asking when play therapy would start for the little one at the Sex Abuse Center. She responded that she was not sure yet about the play therapy and would have to see if the play therapist there would do courtesy sessions with the little one. To date—on May 26, 2016—we have not heard when this will be scheduled.

So we had a nice visit one Sunday evening with the paternal grandparents at the arcade, and then we decided to go to the grocery store. On this day, Aaron and I drove separately, as I had given him a break in the morning to have some personal regrouping time. As we were driving home, I saw someone run across the street with no indication that he or she cared if cars were coming. This person was not crossing at the light and appeared to not care about the two-way traffic in his or her path. As I craned my head to take a closer look, I thought I was going to have a heart attack. It was the girls' mother. What the fuck? Before I could even control myself, I blurted out, "Is that your mother?"

And without missing a beat, the little one responded, "Yup, her hoodie. That's her." Then it set in, and both girls freaked out: "What is she doing here? She is looking for us. I don't want her coming to our house!"

Shit, neither did I. I did the best I could to put on a calm front, but when I got inside, I immediately called the paternal grandmother, asking what she could be doing in the area. She got back to me within minutes that the mother's boyfriend's mother lived close to us, and the bio mother was out on a pass. Freaking fantastic! Now, I had two little girls on edge, thinking she was going to come kidnap them, and I knew we were near the psycho possible sexual abuser. Just great! *Breathe, Chrissie; you hung out with gang members, drug dealers, and so on. You got this! Calm, for the girls.* So that is what I stayed, and we rationally discussed it, coming up with a safety plan.

This incident brought up all kinds of issues for them. The older one was already having nightmares from when her mother was in a car accident from texting and walking in the road. She shared how angry she was at her mother, because she thought her mother had the baby and couldn't believe she would walk across the street like that. I knew the mother had been alone, but clearly the older one was remembering something that had happened with her little brother. Both girls now did not feel like they were in a safe place. Hell, I didn't even feel like we were in a safe place. I quietly wished I could just move us all far away from all of this to make them feel as at peace, innocent, and childlike as they had been in Florida.

May 15, 2016: The girls and I spotted their biological mother one block from our house on the way home from the grocery store. We talked through the sighting and told them to let us know if she comes to the door, as the girls appeared panicked and upset when they saw her, stating, "She's looking for us. I don't want her coming to our house." We were calm in our discussion with the girls, but we did e-mail all workers involved, as it was unexpected to see her that close to our home.

Of course, we got no response from anyone but the therapist, who shared our horror and trepidation with this incident, adding that she felt we handled the whole experience very well.

May 16, 2016: The outpatient mental health program called us and shared that they were unable to get in touch with the state worker after they had left a message. They needed documentation of guardianship in order for the little one to start the program the following day. We had the guardianship letter, so it was sent over.

May 17, 2016: The little one started the outpatient program at the center. After one day, they determined that her needs were too intensive and recommended her for the morning program where one parent will need to be in attendance. We are willing to work our schedule around this program in order to get the little one the help that she needs.

That week during the Thursday visit, which Aaron dutifully took both girls to, I was attempting to take a nap when I was awakened by a phone call from the head of our agency. She shared that she had gotten copied and I was getting a response from the second-in-charge of social services as a response from my communication with the senator. Clearly flabbergasted and without words, she conveyed that our agency wanted to support us and be in on the meeting. She shared that these types of meetings almost never occurred, so it was lucky that this person was reaching back out to me, and she told me to take a deep breath and let the agency respond. I professionally indicated that I wasn't going to be censored, to which she responded that they wanted to represent my concerns and that it was news to her that there had been a recommendation from medical professionals to stop visitation. She assured me that she would take the lead on responding.

When I read the response from the person from social services, I was beyond agitated. She had launched into a spiel about how fostering to adopt was not for everyone. Way to miss the fucking issue! I waited for the head of my agency to respond as she indicated she would. As an administrator, I reiterate with my personnel that it is professional and an expectation to respond within forty-eight hours. I *hate* not adhering to that. Sure, sometimes I miss e-mails that I need to respond to, as I get about two hundred a day and am human, but for the most part, I try to maintain the forty-eight-hour rule. Four days later, there was still nothing from my agency, so I reached out. When I got approval to respond, I of course highlighted the issues I intended to discuss. The head of the agency was pissed. She indicated that this was not the tone we wanted to send. I called her to discuss and explained that, as a leader, I wouldn't want to be blindsided. I gave her an out, stating that if she wasn't going to support me, she didn't have to be there, and I had responded because she hadn't. She replied that she was out of the office that Friday and for the weekend. She was going to get to it first thing. Sure. Excuse after excuse was all I had heard. I was so exhausted from it. Don't claim to advocate if you're not going to. Throughout the time of having the girls, I had learned that these workers in this field don't seem to take communication on Fridays or over the weekend. I really wish I could have that prerogative, but I always find it necessary even when I'm recovering from surgery to respond within forty-eight hours, so this was something I didn't understand.

Finally, after a lot of back and forth, the meeting was set for May 31, after Memorial Day. Of course, my agency wanted to have a meeting prior to that to review my communication. Great, another meeting, another communication. Keep in mind, along with the hellish weekly visitation and the deterioration of the girls as a result, I was still documenting weekly logs. Aaron was still doing therapy twice a week as well, along with monthly psychiatry and anything else that came up in between, all while trying to maintain some realm of family normalcy with expected routines at home.

We were heading out of town to Disney for a four-day-weekend celebration for Aaron's sister's graduation. I had taken two days off work. The girls were thrilled, as they had never imagined they would be able to take this once-in-a-lifetime trip. Aaron's parents had graciously footed the bill, and we would be staying in an amazing eight-bedroom house with them, his sisters, and their friends. It included a private theater and pool. We were all so excited. Of course, in the airport I checked my e-mail to see a ridiculous request from our agency from the state's head, whom we would be meeting with, requesting our home study due to her need to "understand how they responded to questions having to do with willingness and ability to support birth parents and a plan of reunification, what their motivation to foster was, and how they have managed infertility issues." My first reaction was "What the fuck?" My second reaction was "What does that even mean?" My third reaction was to leave the girls in Aaron's care and hop on the damn phone to our agency's supervisor. This certainly felt like some form of retaliation to me, and like hell was I going to give them access to our in-depth home study.

So from the airport terminal, I called to find out what was going on. When I finally got the supervisor on the phone, I asked if we had to comply with this request. She said we did not, and she didn't think the girls could be taken away as a result. Didn't think, great. She as always was a wealth of knowledge. Either way, I knew I would need to contact an attorney. I guessed this would not be a restful break like I thought. But we were boarding, so I put it on the back burner, texting contacts quickly to reach out to attorneys and focusing on the girls' happiness, safety, and comfort as they went on our second destination trip with us.

When we got there, we immediately headed to Disney World, meeting the family and getting our day passes. The girls were thrilled but exhausted and hungry. It wasn't long until the little one had a meltdown, and we had to go our separate way to conquer the hunger and get them settled. We finally arrived at the house, and it was beyond spectacular. I loved seeing the girls' reactions to everything: wonder, amazement, happiness, and childlike excitement. The minute the little one saw the pool, she was rushing to change into her bathing suit and begging for Aaron to go out and get goggles. He complied, because, oh my God, did she make her cute face when she asked. So throughout the weekend we gave the girls the trip of their little lives. We went to Universal Studios, explored each part of the theme park over two days, stopped in gift shops, and got the girls a wide variety of gifts, food, and other memorabilia. On our third day, Aaron's parents once again splurged on all of us, taking us to Disney World. We traipsed through every part of the park we could explore that didn't have long lines. Light-saber wands, princess hats, and princess dolls were all items the girls got that day. They were so happy. It was so great to see them enjoying this experience, taking it all in, and bonding with the older girls in the family. It was also nice to have other people around to get a break. When you're a foster parent, the only option is to send the kids away for respite care, which is a night or two with another licensed foster-care couple within the agency. You can't have family members watch the kids without going through almost the entire, detailed, and lengthy certification process. We had never wanted to send the girls out, because we didn't want to do that to them. So we just endured the exhaustion and parented as best we could, taking full advantage of Sunday school and Girl Scout opportunities where we could get short-term relief.

In between theme parks, I had digitally communicated with a fellow advocate who also had her own agency and was an educational-law consultant. I had the attorney whom I had previously met with, but I needed an attorney who would be able to stand by my side and stand up for my cause in a room where we would be outnumbered. The last day of our trip, in between trying to give the girls the attention, love, and support for them to have an amazing vacation, I got yet another e-mail from our agency's supervisor. She now stated that the state department demanded we take down all social-media pictures of the girls. Unbelievable. Now, I really felt as though we were being attacked. We had never received any training in regard to this. Not to mention that I had been the one filling out forms at school consenting to the girls' pictures being published in the yearbook. Did this extend to that as well? Also, I had the permission of the paternal grandparents, who in the beginning I was told were their legal guardians. It felt like just another assault in a war the state was now waging with us.

I took a break from the girls and got on the phone with the supervisor, because this was how I wanted to spend the last day of what was supposed to be a vacation. I shared how I felt like we were being attacked. She said to take the photos down, but that we had not done anything wrong, and she was drafting a letter to the state department sharing that. She also shared that they were going to be amending their training and foster-care handbook as a result. Yeah, you think? I vented my frustrations at feeling like we were being attacked and did not need this in our lives when we were only trying to care for two amazing little girls but instead were being treated like criminals. She agreed and only offered her support. I told her I had the grandparents' permission on behalf of the girls' biological father. I respected his decision to not come back into the girls' lives and mess it up, as he knew he was a drug addict and could not take care of them. He wanted them with us, because he knew we could give them a chance at a happy, healthy life. After I shared our plight via text with the grandmother, she quickly got on the phone to get the biological father's permission and drafted an e-mail, which I sent to our agency, granting permission for the photos. Of course our agency said it wasn't enough, because they couldn't determine it was authentic and from the biological father. Uh, he was homeless and had no access to a computer. So we had to take down all our wonderful, happy photos where we looked like a family. Each time I hit delete, I felt like someone was stabbing me in the heart. The writing was on the wall, and I knew it was just a matter of time until we would lose the girls. I never could have prepared myself, though, for how horrific and shady the separation from them would be. I just could have never contemplated the cruel, true nature of the giant of a system we were up against.

I finally heard from the attorney recommended by my advocate friend. She sounded very sympathetic and felt that we had a justifiable case, but did not feel as though she was experienced enough in the field to be the one who took it on. She really felt I needed someone who was well versed at dealing with the state, specifically in the area of foster care, and gave me several recommendations, all of whom I followed up with immediately. The day after we returned, I heard back from the most respected one. He quickly listened to my story and bluntly told me to not go in with all the righteous indication I had, because "people within this system are petty people who like to lord their power over others. Go in humble." He wanted me to postpone the meeting in order for him to attend at an hourly rate of $450. I shared that I felt as though I had a sufficient case timeline and would follow up with him if needed afterward.

I had never worked as hard as I did on documentation prior to trying to outline this case in an objective way that lacked emotion and just stated facts. With all my responsibilities, it was something I had to make time for and did. I had to make the case for the best interest of these girls. I loved them. I needed them to be OK, or else what was all of this for? I rocked at documentation. Surely I could make the head of the program see the injustice within this case. Once I got my things together, I had my team of school professionals review it. I needed them to be my anchor ensuring this was not just me and that I had valid concerns. All agreed with me that I did and that this case was unbelievable. I dutifully sent the case timeline to my agency in preparation for our meeting. The head of the agency thought it was very well written and had only a couple of suggestions. When I asked if this case was unusual, I was shocked at the other supervisor's response that the only thing abnormal was my level of advocacy. When I asked how it turned out for most foster kids within their program, I was shocked to hear that same supervisor say they didn't know, because after those kids left their program, they very rarely had any idea what happened to them. That was a far different picture than they had painted in the training. Was I the anomaly here? Maybe I was the one with the wrong perspective. Everyone, including the state, our agency, and hell, even the girls' attorney, seemed nonchalant that this was just the way foster-care cases went. That all the behaviors are a result of the fact that they're foster children, and it's OK, because this is the system. Was I the one that was wrong? As I wiped the tears, listened to the horrific screams and recounting of their night terrors, and instituted intervention after intervention so my little five-year-old did not slip into a dissociative state where she would go catatonic for periods of time, or demonstrate a multitude of emotions in a thirty-second span, or get violent as a result of visitation, I didn't think so.

We were all in agreement for once that I should send the case timeline to the head of social services prior to the meeting. So that is exactly what I did, adding to my e-mail a humane line about having a good weekend. You have seen most of the communication indicated in the timeline above, but below is the rest.

Our Concerns for DSS	Family Law Annotated Code and/or DHR Policy #/Statement	Our Case	Proposed Resolutions for Our Case Along with Future Cases
Lack of Planning/Logistics	Policy SSA-CW #15-18/ The purpose of supervised visits is to ensure the child's physical and emotional safety during contact with parents. In situations where supervised visitation is needed, the local department shall provide a safe and child/family friendly environment for visitation. In situations where supervised visitation is needed, the local department shall provide a safe and child/family friendly environment for the visitation	-2/29: The little one was locked in a cabinet by her sister multiple times on a supervised visit with mom-mom at DSS -No room available or set up prior to any icebreaker, visitation that we've observed or for the Family Meeting. As a result, of DSS workers attempting to scramble around to find a room and worker to watch the children, inappropriate behaviors occurred along with exposure to family members as well as potential abusers.	When setting up a visitation, icebreaker or Family meeting, ensure that there is an available room and worker to watch the children. A sign out sheet of rooms would be helpful in assisting workers along with available to staff who can watch the children with appropriate toys. This can be done digitally along with via a hard copy sign out sheet by the room. Do not indicate childcare will be available if it has not already been set up with an assigned worker/location

Our Concerns for DSS	Family Law Annotated Code and/or DHR Policy #/Statement	Our Case	Proposed Resolutions for Our Case Along with Future Cases
Lack of Implementation of Ground Rules in Family Meetings	SSA # 10-08/ Supervisors shall assume the primary responsibility for family engagement and teaming. The facilitator shall manage time during the meeting. The meetings may last between 1-2 hours. The meeting locations and times shall be conducive to ensuring the participation of the parent or legal guardian and as many team members as possible. The facilitator shall confirm with all team members. The FTM shall assess whether any safety precautions need to be arranged. The facilitator shall have an emergency plan in the event that unforeseen threats to safety arise during the meeting. Special consideration must be given to screen cases to minimize potential risk for further trauma to victims of sexual abuse and domestic violence.	Our FTDM: Facilitator did not confirm with us. We were not told who would be in attendance. Had we been told, we could have discussed safety precautions as well as encounters that could re-traumatize the little one. During the meeting, the biological mother yelled "Fuck your ground rules" and walked out. Additionally, she displayed a lot of hostility and anger towards us without being redirected in any way. She also kept discussing her issues and talking about herself like the topic of the meeting was to get her treatment which caused the meeting to be extended for over 3 hours.	Ensure that all team members receive written notification via an official letter or notice of the FTDM meeting stating the time, location, participants and purpose of the meeting. Offer conducive times for all members and explain if they are unable to attend, they can send a report. Ask if there are any concerns with potential safety and/or exposure to the children to avoid situations that could expose the children in care to additional trauma. Discuss potential consequences with all team members for not following "ground rules" as you are establishing ground rules so expectations are clear and any team member who feels attacked or unsafe understands how to proceed if needed.

Our Concerns for DSS	Family Law Annotated Code and/or DHR Policy #/Statement	Our Case	Proposed Resolutions for Our Case Along with Future Cases
Lack of Follow Through without prompting		See documentation of unreturned calls, e-mails and follow up on issues concerning the girls in regards to scheduling in the case timeline.	Train DSS workers on professional courtesy and responding to communication within a set timeline. Then, communicate that timeline to the families who work with DSS representatives. In the educational system, we train teachers to respond to all communication via phone or e-mail within 24-48 hours with an understanding that they will not communicate on holidays, weekends, scheduled breaks or over the summer. This is a set expectation that is communicated with all stakeholders. Also, train DSS staff to not respond to issues of unavailability by stating that they have too large of a caseload.

Our Concerns for DSS	Family Law Annotated Code and/or DHR Policy #/Statement	Our Case	Proposed Resolutions for Our Case Along with Future Cases
Re-traumatization of the little one through the DSS processes	*Md. FAMILY LAW Code Ann. § 5-525* (e) Reasonable efforts. -- (1) Unless a court orders that reasonable efforts are not required under § 3-812 of the Courts Article or § 5-323 of this title, reasonable efforts shall be made to preserve and reunify families: (i) prior to the placement of a child in an out-of-home placement, to prevent or eliminate the need for removing the child from the child's home; and (ii) to make it possible for a child to safely return to the child's home. (2) In determining the reasonable efforts to be made and in making the reasonable efforts described under paragraph (1) of this subsection, **the child's safety and health shall be the primary concern.** (3) Reasonable efforts to place a child for adoption or with a legal guardian may be **made concurrently with the reasonable efforts described under paragraph (1) of this subsection.** (f) Development of a permanency plan. -- (1) In developing a permanency plan for a child in an out-of-home placement, the local department shall give **primary consideration to the best interests of the child,** including consideration of both in-State and out-of-state placements. The local department shall **consider the following factors in determining the permanency plan that is in the best interests of the child:** **(i) the child's ability to be safe and healthy in the home of the child's parent;** **(ii) the child's attachment and emotional ties to the child's natural parents and siblings;** **(iii) the child's emotional attachment to the child's current caregiver and the caregiver's family;** **(iv) the length of time the child has resided with the current caregiver;** **(v) the potential emotional, developmental, and educational harm to the child if moved from the child's current placement; and** **(vi) the potential harm to the child by remaining in State custody for an excessive period of time.**	Biological mother convicted of the following: 10/14/15: -Child Abuse-second degree -Second Degree Assault 5/14/15: -Confinement of unattended child The little one had not seen her biological mother in over a year when visitation started at DSS. Prior to that she had not lived with her biological mother since the age of 3. The little one does not call her mom, "mom" but instead by her middle name. See prior documentation of the little one being locked in a cabinet and potential exposure to mom's boyfriend (alleged abuser) at the FTDM. Since visitation started with the biological mother, her mental state has increasingly deteriorated. Documented concerns from each visit have included: -an increase in sexualized behavior (taking naked selfies, kissing boys, sitting in their laps, licking the private areas of stuffed animals) -acting out domestic violence with dolls -increase in extreme dissociation -increase in violent behaviors -significant regression to acting like a baby particularly at the age of 3 -self injurious behaviors Recommendations of therapist and psychiatrist ignored for the little one's visitation with her mother. She now has a 504 plan within the school setting. The IOP at the mental health institution has explained that her needs are so intensive she needs a morning day program where a parent is able to stay with her for the duration. She is currently on the wait list.	Set a court date to reduce visitation to at least monthly visitation with biological mother for the little one and/or stop visitation based on professional's recommendations that work with her until she is in a more stable mental state. When she is in a more stable mental state, slowly reintegrate visitation with biological parent per recommendations from all doctors working with her. Since the biological mother has expressed that she will sign all of her rights over to the little one's paternal step-grandmother, schedule an earlier permanency plan meeting for her. With the little one's extensive behavioral needs, she requires a home in which she will have adult(s) that are capable of keeping up with her appointments, therapy, interventions, etc. Consider separating the girls. Provide the compelling reason as to why it has been determined that termination of parental rights would not be in the little one's best interests.

Our Concerns for DSS	Our Case
Concern for retaliation	Prior to sending a request to the senator to speak to someone in regards to our concerns, no issues were brought to our attention verbally or in written form in regards to concerns with the care we were providing as foster parents.
	Since this meeting has been scheduled, we have had a unique request for our home study: "understand how they responded to questions having to do with willingness and ability to support birth parents and a plan of reunification, what their motivation to foster was, and how they have managed infertility issues."
	We have also received notification to take down photos in regards to Facebook pictures. This policy was never reviewed with us by our DSS caseworker. It was stated in a letter sent to our agency that we require biological consent for photos in which we have gotten via the paternal grandfather for the biological father of the girls.
	Concerns in regards to us staying for visits with grandparents were conveyed to our agency but never shared with us. The DSS worker was aware we were staying for visitation. (see above in case timeline 3/11 and 4/1 along with in the below table)

DSS Concerns with Us	Our Case	Proposed Resolutions Moving Forward
- An understanding of the reunification process and the rights of the birth families - Not respecting and honoring the birth family and the children's relationship with them Premature interest in adoption	See previous documentation. Had clear expectations been established along with a visitation plan within 3 business days of receiving this case, we would not have been introduced to the girls and started our relationship as potential adoptive parents. We also would not have taken this case. We have established positive relationships with the paternal grandparents, biological father, and even the maternal grandmother (to the point that we are have respectful interactions with mom-mom, communicate on a weekly basis and call monthly.) We have maintained professionalism during interactions with the biological mother even though she has not given us the same courtesy. We understand that the primary purpose of visitation is to maintain the parent/child attachment while reducing the child's sense of abandonment and preserving the sense of family for a child residing in an out of home placement.	- Outline a clear follow up of the plan for visitation, proceeding with an earlier court hearing for the little one based on recommendations from the professionals working with her. - Provide us with a timeline for the earliest that reunification could occur along with the timeline for a request for guardianship to be returned to the paternal grandparents. If other family members (paternal step grandmother or mom-mom) are interested in keeping the oldest one, consider this placement option and separating the girls due to their own needs that require constant and excessive attention. There is a lack of a bond between them as siblings and they have a detrimental impact on one another. - Have supervised visitation alternate between our agency and the state. Help us to understand what a visit that goes "very well" looks like and inform us of anything that is being said that could trigger the girls. A lot of discussion in regards to future promises, money and checks have been discussed with the girls by biological mom at each visit from what the girls have shared with us. DSS has not disclosed discussions that have occurred.

DSS Concerns with Us	Our Case	Proposed Resolutions Moving Forward
Staying for unsupervised visits with the grandparents	We asked for guidelines in regards to these visits on 3/11 and were only told: bi-weekly and in the community. On 4/1, the DSS caseworker e-mailed indicating she was aware of us staying for visits. She set guidelines which we have adhered to on these visits. No follow up ever occurred until we reached out to share concerns with the Senator in regards to DSS.	We still have not been given a clear directive on whether we should stay or not stay for visits, so as of 5/28, we are not staying for these community visits.

Foster-Care Process Considerations for Change

We would respectfully like DSS to consider advocating to amend the system to include cases that have been within "in home services." We would like those time considerations that kids in foster care have spent to be taken into account and combined.

So many things within the foster care system are currently on a case by case basis, yet there is a blanket 15 months for attempting to terminate parental rights. These girls have been in an alternate side of DSS since 10/14 and were already placed in foster care for one weekend in September 2015. That is 16 months in the system prior to officially entering foster care and staying longer than a weekend. That is also almost 21 months that biological parents have had to make progress and get their children back in this case. State money would be reduced greatly if this could be considered and factored in when cases are switched over to foster care from another department.

Throughout our dealings with DSS in this process, we have heard from multiple people within a professional capacity such as attorneys and workers within other agencies who have shared that most of the time DSS workers are not present, cancel at the last minute and are not consistent with following the same protocol. The perception from the public in regards to DSS is extremely negative. Most people will say that they have heard "horror stories" from multiple sources. In our case, we have been told that we have to watch the little one deteriorate mentally as a result of visitation so it is documented over time. Additionally, we have been told that it is not significant enough and that within the system there is currently a case where a biological parent who hears voices, has mental illness and has threatened to kill her children is currently slated for reunification. Another case that was shared with us by the DSS social worker was that of a biological parent being convicted of murder who got their child back when they got out of prison and now the child is right back in the foster care system. Currently, there is a lawsuit in South Carolina where the following is stated: "There's got to be accountability when longstanding systemic problems, like a severe lack of mental health services, gross overreliance on institutions and high caseloads, continue to harm innocent children" (http://thinkprogress.org/health/2015/01/14/3611475/south-carolina-dss-lawsuit/). MD DSS needs to consider this statement, article and the impact their employees are having on people they encounter by presenting these same concerns when referring to a lack of follow through due to their caseloads, as well as the perception they are contributing to where there is "horror story after horror story within DSS."

Train DSS workers and families in the area of dealing with PTSD. Instead of stating repeatedly that all children in foster care display these behaviors, take the PTSD symptoms on a case by case basis deferring to recommendations of healthcare professionals working with those children in order to foster each child's healthiest mental state. PTSD in high doses of adversity affect kids' brains structure and function and the way their DNA is read and transcribed. The following is an outstanding resource:

https://www.ted.com/talks/nadine_burke_harris_how_childhood_trauma_affects_health_across_a_lifetime?language=en

The Adverse Childhood Experience (ACE) Questionnaire is referred to in the above video. Kids with a high ACE score have the following statistics with an ACE score of 4 or more:

- *2 ½ times more likely to develop diseases such as hepatitis*
- *4 ½ times more likely to develop depression*
- *12 times more likely to take their own life*

If the little one were to take this questionnaire today, her ACE score would be 9.

When I got a response from her within the next couple of hours stating that "admittedly she had to chuckle when she read about the suggestions for correspondence due to the recent difficulty she had with the school system I was affiliated with," I knew this was going to be an even rougher meeting than I had anticipated. I knew my concerns were going to fall on deaf ears. A part of me just wanted to give up, to not even show up. This was all so emotionally draining, mentally depleting. Aaron and I were in a rough patch. We were going around the clock twenty-four hours a day with work, the girls, the visits, the documentation, and so on. It was hard enough to just be parents. Jesus, it was the hardest job I had ever done, but to factor in all these other minutiae was beyond frustrating. I couldn't help but wonder, again, why it felt like a punishment when all we wanted to do was keep these girls safe, love them, cherish them, keep them from harm, and give them a permanent home. As much as I wanted to run away, I knew I had to fight—it was for them.

Aaron and I decided during this time that we were going to proceed with the IVF process that we had decided upon and even set up the day we had gotten the call for the girls. I set up my appointment, and the day I had my blood work done was the day of the meeting. We had talked with the girls about our decision to have a baby, and they were elated. The little one thought that, the minute I went to the doctor, I would be pregnant. The minute I got home, she said: "Is there a baby in your tummy, Mommy?" She could be so preciously innocent when she wasn't plagued with the traumatic thoughts that rotated around her mind.

On the day of the meeting, I had taken off. Both Aaron and I took the little one to her therapy session that morning. We read a book together as she melted in my arms. The therapist was in awe at how much she had grown since being in our care. It was a moment I would look back on and cherish, despite being saddened at its memory. We all had a wonderful weekend at my mom's swim club. I had the pictures to prove it, but they remained hidden in my phone, as I all too painfully knew that Big Brother State Department was watching.

On the way to the meeting, I got a call from the fertility center. Everything was good to go to start the IVF process. I reveled at the timing. I had started with IVF in mind when I got the call for the girls. Now, as it appeared my time with them was coming to an end, IVF was the viable option again. We met up with our agency's representative, the supervisor, the supervisor under her, and our social worker. I felt as though I was a criminal being taken to death row as we checked in with security and took the dreaded maze through the corridor of offices down to the disgusting conference room where we had the unpleasant FTDM meeting. The state worker, her supervisor, and a little troll-like woman with unruly curly hair and glasses sat next to them. She was not what I had expected at all, looking like a younger version of Rhea Perlman, but she definitely had a hardened, strong presence about her, so I knew she was the head of the program. She introduced herself, and we made small talk as pleasantly as we could considering the circumstances. As I commented on her reply about the lack of follow-up within my educational system, trying to break the ice and be helpful by directing her to whom she could have spoken to, she said that at least schools had secretaries who answered the phone. Their department had received a cut in funding, so they didn't have any support. She then basically bashed our agency for being private by saying that she wished they had the power to turn cases away, but being public, they didn't have that option. Oh, this was going to be a really fun meeting. We were off to a grand start!

She explained that the girls' attorney was on the way. I said that we needed to leave within an hour and a half in order to pick up the girls from the bus stop. She distributed probably the saddest attempt at an agenda paper I had ever seen—a title with three dashes of topics under it. She started by saying that although there had been many meetings already, we were back with another one to address what she felt like was a misunderstanding of the system. She started off by quoting the parable from "The Elephant and the Blind Men." With the amount of times she interrupted herself and considering I had no visual in front of me as she was quoting this, I really had no idea what she was fucking talking about. But I felt Aaron tense up, his hostility building within his body, which rarely happened, so I knew it wasn't a good moral to this story and was painting a rough picture of us. After the meeting I did further research on the tale, and this is what I found:

The parable of the blind men and the elephant is used to illustrate how biases can blind us, preventing us from seeking a more complete understanding on the nature of things. It is often used as a warning against the promotion of absolute truths.

The parable went something like this:

In a distant village, a long time ago, there lived six blind men. One day the villagers announced, "Hey, there is an elephant in the village today."

They had never seen or felt an elephant before and so decided, "Even though we would not be able to see it, let us go and feel it anyway." And thus they went down to the village to touch and feel the elephant to learn what animal this was and they described it as follows:

"Hey, the elephant is a pillar," said the first man who touched his leg.

"Oh, no! it is like a rope," argued the second after touching the tail.

"Oh, no! it is like a thick branch of a tree," the third man spouted after touching the trunk.

"It is like a big hand fan" said the fourth man feeling the ear.

"It is like a huge wall," sounded the fifth man who groped the belly.

"It is like a solid pipe," said the sixth man with the tusk in his hand.

They all fell into heated argument as to who was right in describing the big beast, all sticking to their own perception. A wise sage happened to hear the argument, stopped and asked them "What is the matter?" They said, "We cannot agree to what the elephant is like."

The wise man then calmly said, "Each one of you is correct; and each one of you is wrong. Because each one of you had only touched a part of the elephant's body. Thus you only have a partial view of the animal. If you put your partial views together, you will get an idea of what an elephant looks like."

Although the parable's function is to call attention to a lack of objectivity and consideration of other approaches and perspectives when trying to understand the nature of things, we do have to warn that not all perspectives are equally valid, and even valid arguments are not necessarily equally sound. (https://wildequus.org/2014/05/07/sufi-story-blind-men-elephant/)

So mainly she wanted us to know that our arguments had no validity, and basically, we were wrong. She proceeded to dismiss my care for the girls, reiterating with blunt, matter-of-fact honesty that they were not my children. And it was like "I went on four dates and called a caterer." As she went through the traditional spiel of how fostering was "shared parenting," I cut her off, stating, "And that is exactly why we didn't want to foster. We were in this as a preadoptive resource." In response, she basically scolded us for going with a private agency, promoting her own adoption-resource agencies within the state's system and stating how within their training they have an attorney who explains that fostering to adopt takes a minimum of two to three years. Oh, and there really wasn't such a thing as a preadoptive resource. Not only did she scold us but she also seriously called out our agency, stating that if this was our intent that was shared from the beginning, we probably wouldn't have passed the state's version of the home study.

Finally, the supervisor spoke up, sharing that they used the same home study. But she was quickly shot down again, with the head of the state indicating that they really needed to "step up their communication." I couldn't disagree with that; however, it was sobering to see our agency, who had proclaimed to be the advocates above advocates, get put in their place so easily, like they were puppies who had just been scolded by their master. Finally, the attorney walked in. She had no notes and a reluctant look on her face. Even though I had been the one to communicate with her in regard to the meeting, I knew she had to be on the side of the state. She was a no name attorney that no other attorney I had consulted with knew, so my impression was that she was pretty low on the totem pole and had to maintain the status quo in order to keep her job.

The meeting continued in a tense fashion. The state head of the department continued by saying that the girls knew we didn't want them to have visits, and it was preventing them to be able to move forward in a healthy manner with the reunification plan. They brought up how Aaron had said he didn't want them to go on a visit. Keep in mind this was on a date when the social worker hadn't let us know the visit was scheduled, so both girls were surprised and screaming they didn't want to go while clinging to Aaron's legs. What the hell are you supposed to do in a situation like that? Be an unfeeling robot of a human being and shove them out the door? She went on to say that "they don't chase down medical records," so unless the therapist wanted to come testify—at which point I interrupted and said, "She would; just let us know when." That threw her off her memorized speech for a second.

When it came out that the social worker had not followed up with us about the play therapy or responded, the worker muttered a halfhearted apology. When I shared that communication had been like this throughout our stint as foster parents, the head of them said, "OK, well, she apologized. I'm not going to get into who struck John." Again, I had no idea what the fuck that meant, but I knew she didn't want to own up to anything. This was something I didn't understand. I myself was a leader and had worked under both great and awful leaders. One of the most human things you can do to alleviate tension with someone who feels justified in his or her complaint is to own up to something, apologize, and be genuine with that apology. I knew that was not going to happen in this setting.

Then, to add fuel to the fire, the supervisor of the state worker said that the forensic interview had come back inconclusive anyway and for the little one to get play therapy was not necessary. I brought up the notes from the FTDM meeting—you know, where this same woman had suggested that the additional play therapy occur at their center in conjunction with the therapy from her trauma professional—but I was dismissed. Then, she asked the girls' attorney to address the legal concerns. Of course, she didn't have any statutes or legal notes in front of her, so when I asked about case law, she couldn't answer my questions or basis for arguments with any valid points. She just referred me to a resource. Basically, what she had to add was that within the law, for termination of parental rights to be considered earlier than the timeline they were adhering to for *all* cases, it had to be something really egregious and a prior conviction of second-degree child abuse wasn't even close.

Aaron was doing his best to not boil over at that point, and when the head of the state asked him why he looked perplexed, he stated that he was. He also asked what could be considered egregious. For example, did someone have to cut up the child into pieces? Would that be egregious enough? No one could answer that. They just said to look it up, that this case wouldn't even come close, and the level of egregiousness was considered on a case-by-case basis. If you're processing this like I was, it surely didn't make sense. For termination of parental rights to be considered, it has to be egregious, but there is no set definition. So it is reviewed on a case-by-case basis, but the protocol is to follow a specific timeline for all cases. Was I crazy? This made absolutely no sense to me.

Then, to illustrate what a visit looks like when it goes "very well," this head bitch distributed photos from a visit with the biological mom. Now, these photos could have been taken within thirty seconds. She said that she came to observe the visit because of all the fuss I had made, and the visit as illustrated went very well. I got the timeline of her visit straight and asked, "Oh, was this the visit when the mother gave them water bottles with a strange-smelling liquid inside?" She took a beat and ignored my question. They played a game, and the little one was sitting in her mom's lap. As I looked through the photos, I just felt as though I had been stabbed in the heart.

They indicated that the red flags were there in this case, but that it would take two to three years to even move forward with terminating parental rights. And until then, they knew the mom would relapse, but they were going to assist her with working the program so that she could get her kids back, even if it meant they all lived in one room. Because they don't take kids from the lower class and give them to the middle class. Middle class. It was like we were being ostracized because we had the means to take care of them. She furthered revealed her bias against our position in the class system by stating that foster parents already had an advantage over biological parents, because they were able to give more. I had never felt so criticized and devalued for making it to my standing. I had hung out in the ghetto. I remember scraping a loaf of bread together and using the crusts to scrape the peanut butter out of the jar because that was all the food in my house. Yet I was the bad guy, because I didn't have food stamps and would never think of selling them to get money for drugs. She didn't go back to my concerns and didn't address one issue I had brought to her attention. She just continued on her self-righteous rant, highlighting a vague percentage about her success rates. With a sadistic look on her face and a smirk, she said, "Most people say I'm sending kids home to die." But her research and data, as she shared, indicated that reunification was the best plan. I guess because they don't have time to chase down medical records, they wouldn't know the drastic mental or emotional ramifications to the child.

I was never going to win this. I was so sick of fighting. These people sitting around this table honestly did not feel that there was anything wrong with this process, and in my heart and soul, after seeing the effects on these girls I loved, all I could see was the detriment it caused them. I told them we could no longer continue. I could sense their relief. They were finally going to be done with my advocacy and with us. I broke down in tears. I couldn't hold it in anymore. Whether they thought it was right or not, I did love these girls. I mentioned that as I made them all promise that they would look out for them. I also told them that when the time came for rights to be terminated, they should remember that they had two people who loved those girls more than anything. We talked about a timeline for them leaving their care. I had said that I would've liked to take the little one to her treatment in the intensive outpatient program. We agreed on four to six weeks. They thanked us, happy that "we weren't saying for them to get out within a couple of days." I left there completely devastated. If I ever saw that place again, it would be too soon. I just wanted to wash away the whole experience, as I felt so vile at having to interact with their level of self-righteousness in the injustice of the system for the kids in their care.

I was sobbing and having difficulty catching my breath as Aaron drove the twenty minutes home. He was trying to comfort me as best he could, but he too was mentally drained and emotionally destroyed. I knew the girls could not see me like this, so I had to get myself together. But where to? Where do you go when you feel like your whole world has just crumbled? I couldn't go to school, and I looked a hot mess. So I had Aaron pull over on the side of the road into a parking lot, called my secretary, and had her get my mom. When my mom got on the phone, I was so hysterical I couldn't even get words out that made sense. The only thing I could manage to say was that I had failed, because that is exactly how I felt. Like I had failed those girls. I had given this my all. Should I have just taken the check and stood by, watching what in my opinion was injustice continue? That's just not who I was, and it would never be. But I had lost, and now I was going to lose the only babies I had ever known. All I could imagine was the state worker coming to pick them up, ripping them out of our arms with all their things in tow. I was in the midst of a horrible panic attack. I hadn't cried that hard since my stepfather passed away, and my eyes had welted up, all sore, bloodshot, and devoid of light.

Like all parents do when you have responsibilities and little ones depending on you, I got myself together, fixed my face, and went home to try to cherish my last moments with them. We all got changed and went to the pool. I wished I could float it all away. I just tried to savor every movement, every interaction with them. After we got home and got settled, we sat them down and talked to them about the change. We explained that they would be going to another foster family but that it wasn't because we didn't love or want them. We tried as best we could to relieve their worried minds and answer their questions. I was so depleted. And yet I had to keep some semblance of stability for them, so that is what I did, trying to keep our routines consistent.

After we had gotten them tucked in bed, I was going to turn off the light, when all of a sudden I felt woozy, the room started spinning, and before I knew it, I was passed out on the ground. Aaron was over top of me, debating if he needed to call an ambulance, calculating my heart rate and blood pressure. I just tried to breathe. My body was so weak. I knew it was just a severe panic attack. Once I got up and was able to get into bed, my mind was at unrest. I tossed and turned all night, wondering if it was in our best interest to have a four-to-six-week time frame or if it would destroy me to spend more time with them and then have them ripped away from us. I was especially concerned because they had their weekly visit coming up. After our horrific experience at that place, I knew Aaron and I could no longer drive to that building. The next day I e-mailed our worker to ask how long the timeline would be as well as to share that we no longer wanted contact with the state. My subtext was that our agency needed to pick up the responsibilities for taking the girls to and from visits so that we would not have to endure further emotional trauma. I got a brief message that she would follow up with her supervisor.

The next day in the midst of my busy team-meeting schedule, the supervisor called me. I asked if they had a resource for the girls, as in another placement. She said that they didn't and that they had just filed our official resignation of the case that day, so we had thirty days minimum left. When I asked about a timeline, she said she didn't know. She started to talk about us bringing the girls to a picnic so they could meet other foster parents, to which I basically responded that if she thought I was going to help someone else take them, she should think again. She said that there was no way we could not communicate with the state, because technically they were the legal guardians. The underlying factor was that this supervisor also had two other jobs and didn't want to be bothered with this case, because our agency worker was going on vacation.

She asked if the talk was helpful. I said it was not, because at this point all communication with any agency representative made us feel frustrated. She asked if we were able to continue with their care in the interim, and I replied that we could at least until the end of school, which was two weeks away. Of course, she wanted us to come in for a meeting that day. Our worker would take the girls to the visit, and Aaron would pick them up at the end of the visit from our meeting, so we would have minimal interaction with the state. Having to actually do my job, I was unable to drive all the way to their agency to meet, so I instead joined them on the phone. We continued the conversation in the same manner we had discussed earlier that day, except this time Aaron did more of the talking. I was done. We ended the meeting with nothing more resolved. Our worker, who was going on vacation, told Aaron that she wouldn't be able to assist the next week but wanted to help that night, so she offered to pick up the girls so that Aaron could come home and get a minibreak.

When he got home thirty minutes later, we had just begun to commiserate when he got a text from the worker saying that she was taking them out to dinner to give us more of a break. He texted back thanking her for her generosity. Ten minutes later, the supervisor of our worker, yet not the one in charge of our agency, called. Aaron picked up and stammered, "Hang on; can you say that again while I put you on speaker?" Christ, what now! I had never heard Aaron use that tone before, so I had no idea what to expect. I will never forget the sound of that heartless bitch's voice as she said calmly with pregnant pauses: "Just from our talks earlier, and hearing how done you were, we decided to place them tonight." The statement hung in the air. She repeated it and then stated that we would need to pack a bag for them. Aaron was confused. He asked a couple of questions to clarify, but I knew what it meant. The state had taken them on the visit. Even though this supervisor said it was her call and she would have to live with it, I knew she was a puppet. All I could manage to say to her was, "So we don't even get to say good-bye to them." She said she was working on that. I told her how shady this all was and disconnected.

It was done. Our babies were gone. I had no idea where they were, what they were thinking, or how upset and confused they must be. They thought they were coming home to watch a movie. Instead they were carted off to God knows where with strangers. No one can tell me that was in their best interest, especially for the little one and her PTSD. As Aaron raced around to get what things we could in a bag, I got on the phone. We had to get out of the house. I could not be in this house without them. I called my boss, explained what had occurred, and took off for the next day. Then, I called the hotel I always stayed in when going to the ocean, quickly making a reservation and not caring about the cost. I needed to get out and try to make sense of this. We dropped the girls' sad bags off with our neighbor from New York, who was so pissed at the situation. We hoped she would cuss our agency out when they arrived. In contrast their lack of courtesy with not telling us until after the fact about this horrible transition, Aaron texted instructions as to where the bags could be found. She wrote back asking if we wanted to say anything to the girls. Yes, there was a lot we wanted to say. But not over her phone, not through text, and not this way.

I couldn't believe that our agency, the ones who were supposed to be partners with us and advocates for the children, had been the ones to do this, to end it this way. If they had said at our meeting that an emergency placement was an option, we probably would have gone for it. But no, they had to be cloak-and-dagger. I wondered if it was even a ruse for our worker to take them out to dinner. I knew it probably had been and struggled with the fact that my opinion of her had been that she was a kind, empathetic human being. I didn't understand how I could've been so wrong. The further we drove, the more it sunk in that it was really over. I was no longer a mom to the two girls I had given up my world for. Halfway into our three-and-a-half-hour drive, I found the courage to post on social media about what had happened. So many people had been supporting our plight and praying for us. I owed it to them to share the story. This is what I wrote:

We believed, loved, advocated, fought and lost.

Tonight DSS took the girls out of our care while they were on a visit…without our knowledge. We didn't even get to say good-bye. Every bad thing you've heard about DSS Foster care doesn't even come close to how despicable they are. One quote that will forever resonate from the woman in charge of social services to us was that they are not our children and it was like we went on 4 dates and called a caterer. All that said I know God is greater than any situation or evil. I pray now for him to watch over the 2 beautiful, amazing girls we were blessed to have call us mom and dad for 5 months.

We got over sixty comments from people who were disgusted and wanted to reach out to express their love and support. Somehow it helped ease the sting of the pain, at least a little bit.

CHAPTER 8

There's No Place like IVF

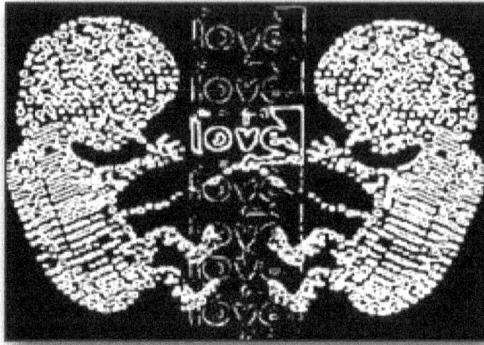

"THEY'RE NOT YOUR CHILDREN. IT's like you went on four dates and called a caterer!" Self-righteous bitch! A month later, and her words still played in my head, rotating like an old broken record. There was so much I wish I had said, like "Yes, you bitch, I actually did call a caterer right away, because I knew my husband was the one after I banged him on the first night. And aren't we supposed to think of them as our children? That's why we were fostering to adopt as a fucking preadoptive resource!" I know; really professional, right? I was wallowing in my feelings. Somehow, as horrible as that woman was, I had managed to maintain my composure and dignity. It was the right move. Anything ignorant I might have said would've fallen on deaf ears. After all, the dismissive nature and overwhelming lack of interest in the case of our girls made all of them so evil and robotic in their own way.

I just kept telling myself it was better this way to be rid of the system. But that didn't stop the ache in my heart for the girls I had come to know and love as my own. My thoughts revolved around them. Were they OK? Fuck, I hoped they were. What had DSS or our agency told them? And my dreams trying to make sense of the whole situation were very tumultuous. Not to mention the deafening silence that surrounded me at home. For five months, I had been "Mommy." My whole world revolved around them from food to activities to their well-being. There was nothing I wouldn't have or didn't do for them while they were in my care, because to me and Aaron, they were our children. Hell, even to the girls, we were their parents. How come no one told us up front we weren't supposed to love them like our own? Where is that on the damn fostering-to-adopt commercials or articles that make it look like a fucking walk in the park? No, they weren't ours. For whatever reason, the state was determined to make their mom a success story. Reunification to a former heroin addict, child abuser. They don't seem to write fairy tales about that.

The other thing that didn't help my mental state was the daily injections I was getting, filled with medication designed to boost my fertility but not a friend of my depression medication. Whether it was the side effects of that or the situation was hard to decipher, it was clear I was depressed.

I felt like an empty shell. A robot going through the daily routine but numb to everything around me. It was very similar to the grieving process I'd endured so many times in my life after the loss of a loved one. For five months, even though they were a tumultuous five months, I had been Mommy. My life had a newfound purpose that revolved around the wants and needs of our two girls. And I had loved every minute of being with them, spoiling them every chance I got. My credit-card bills still had the balance to prove it. For those five months, I felt a type of happiness and purpose in my life I had never known. There was a light in my eyes, an energy in my step no matter how exhausted I was, and a glow in my face. All of that was gone now as I still struggled to make sense of it all.

In the midst of a house filled with clutter, messes, and kids throwing tantrums as well as inexplicably being the pickiest eaters alive, what does every parent wish for? Solitude, quiet—peace. The life you had before them, where you could watch a TV show without animation. When you could drink a beer without a little person asking what that is, or demanding your immediate and constant attention. The ability to leave the house without a frustrating hide-and-seek game with the children's shoes. No matter how many times you put them in a location that you believe to be convenient, one of those fuckers is always missing. This, inevitably, leads to a shoe hunt for the whole family that ends up taking twenty minutes. Actually going to restaurants that you enjoy without having to bargain about whether or not we go to Chuck E. Cheese's. The ability to go to the bathroom or undress in your home without screaming little people barging in or hearing the relentless shouts of "Mom," which get louder and more annoying the more you try to not respond. And sleep, oh my God, sleep. To have even four to six hours of uninterrupted, peaceful sleep would be amazing. These were the things that we had craved in moments of chaos, frustration, and the endless cycle of catering to two of the cutest what felt like dictators. These were the things we were trying to focus on. We had what we tried to think of as "our life back." But the freedom didn't feel as good as we had built it up in our minds. It felt lonely and depressing. The silence was almost mocking, making me feel as though I had dreamed the whole experience.

Over the years I've taken on a personal life motto that aligns with my faith: "Life may knock me down, but it will never knock me out." This situation sure had knocked me down on my ass. Our house, once filled with children's laughter and the pitter-patter of their feet, now lay dormant with a deafening silence that was hard to ignore. As a mom there were moments I had wished for a minute of peace and a somewhat clean house that didn't get overturned within seconds by the child tornado that was our girls. Now I'd give anything to have it all back.

It's better this way, I kept trying to tell myself, continuously losing the endless argument in my mind. *We have our life back. We can sleep, watch TV other than cartoons and TeenNick, eat meals that don't revolve around the picky choices of finicky girls, walk around naked if we want, and drink. We can go out anytime, not having to worry about childcare. Freedom.* I should have been elated, but instead I just felt emptiness and a sickening sinking feeling in my stomach every time I looked around at the bare surroundings that were supposed to be home.

We set our minds to focus on the future: IVF, selling our house as soon as possible, and finally moving to Florida like we had always wanted but had put on hold at the chance of adoption. After everything we had already been through, I wasn't leaving anything to fate with IVF, so when they asked if we wanted the genetic testing, I quickly agreed. It was such a relief when that and my blood work all came back clear. Finally, something was moving at a consistent, positive pace.

—⸎—

I remember some of the trials and tribulations we ended up facing while trying to get this accomplished. We weren't necessarily far from home. Ocean City is only a three-hour drive from Baltimore. The problem was that Chrissie needed to start the IVF process on that day or not at all. Well, at least not for another month. That did not sit well with either of us, and Chrissie, being on the emotional edge for longer than I can remember her being (and she has teetered on that edge for a long time in the past), began to cry. "I don't want to wait another month to start this, Aaron! I can't stand it!"

I understood, in a less direct way, about what was going through her head. Mind you, I have never and will never say that I know definitively what it is like for a woman to feel her biological clock dwindling and the event horizon that is utter infertility quickly coming upon her. I don't know what kind of insanity that would cause in me if our roles were reversed. However, I will also say that I am a rather empathetic person. I am capable of putting myself in other people's shoes better than most. In this case, Chrissie's panic and ensuing emotional tidal wave of despair were not falling on deaf ears. We both got on phones and eventually were able to get in touch with the doctor. After the initial contact with the fertility staff, I told Chrissie to put her cell phone down, and I would handle the rest. The rest included quite a few annoying steps. We had to get the first round of birth control into her *that day*. Unfortunately, the prescription was sent to the pharmacy that we usually go to. This is of course located in our lovely hometown of—you guessed it! Fucking Parkville of fucking Baltimore son of bitching County! So after multiple calls and conversations with the staff of the pharmacy and of the fertility clinic, I somehow was able to get the prescription transferred to a pharmacy in the Ocean City area! How awesome am I? So awesome that when I picked up the prescription, I forgot to take it with me after I paid for it at the register! I drove all the way back to the damn hotel we were staying in, just basking in my own fantastic coordinating skills. Then, as I was getting out of the car, I reached my stupid arm over to the passenger seat, where I stupidly thought I had left the prescription. You know what I found when I placed my dumb fingers on that seat? *Nothing!* I was about to slam my own skull through the windshield. Had I gone through all that and given Chrissie such hope and myself a much-needed confidence boost, only to have it dashed by my own dumb, stupid, idiot brain? I decided, no. No, I will not have come so close to victory only to fail now. It had to be back at the pharmacy. The pills were going to be in that white bag on the counter, I would take them back to my wife, and I would still be the ragged victor. At the end of the day, I was going to be the fucking hero, and no one, not even myself, was going to get in the way!

I drove back to the pharmacy, clutching the steering wheel of our black Kia Soul as if I were white knuckling the reins of a galloping black horse. I sped down the rain-sodden streets at admittedly dangerous speeds, running through lights that had turned yellow for just a little too long by the time I passed through their intersections. Squealing into the parking lot, I felt like I was going in slow motion, action-movie-hero style. I like to think that plumes of smoke spat out from behind my tires as I made the turn into the pharmacy, but that is surely memory theater. I ran inside, my face covered in sweat as I ran to the counter. "Hey!" I said to the cashier from whom I had made the purchase. "I…may have left some—" The girl behind the counter—she couldn't have been older than nineteen and had the expression to match— simply held up that damn white bag, full of the precious tiny pills that might have the beginning of our journey to parenthood. She held it up with a face that clearly judged me, and I felt, in that moment, like a ragged traveler in one of my many fantasy novels, at the end of his first quest. Bereft of spirit, soul torn, body exhausted, but victorious nonetheless.

I drove back to the hotel yet again. The cold sweat that had drenched my face and neck was drying up and leaving me rather parched. As I waited for the elevator, I drank what felt like three gallons of tepid water from a nearby water fountain in an effort to flood the mini-Sahara that was my mouth. The elevator dinged, and I hurriedly wiped the excess water from my face. I nearly collided with a young couple and a baby on the way into the elevator car and felt as though that was an appropriate event to have preceded my perilous journey.

Having reached the floor that Chrissie and I were staying on, I shuffled out of the elevator and made my way down the hall toward our room. The carpet, I noticed, was actually quite plush and lovely. It was weird, the appreciation I had for the little surrounding aspects of the hotel that had escaped me upon our arrival. I remember taking out my key card and inserting it into the slot; my hand was all shaky and sweaty. It took me two or three attempts to get the damn door open. I walked in with the bag, holding what we thought would be the key to our future as parents, held high! Chrissie actually said, "Yay! My hero!" That, at least, made it all worth it. She had a giant smile on her face and looked like someone had actually saved the day for her. I felt pretty damn good too, despite my fuckup. I had fixed the terrible situation that was Chrissie's way-be-gone medicine. And I fixed the problem I myself had caused. I feel like, in that way, I was a hero to my wife and myself. We left on Sunday. We drove home thinking that we were going to be parents, and we were just going to be the absolute best. We had no goddamned clue what type of ride we were in for.

The struggle, in this case, was absolutely goddamned real.

And that, ladies and gentlemen, was only the first in an incredibly long and difficult path that would be our journey through IVF. After everything else that we had been through, there was still so much more to go. If only we had seen it then, just what it was to embark on this endeavor. The amount of commitment, energy, and sacrifice to be able to do something that really should have been a relatively easy thing. But for Chrissie and me, nothing comes easy. That was a theme of our lives even before we met. And I didn't care one bit about taking the hard road if it meant that I got to do it with my wife.

~ᴄ

The month had flown by since the girls were ripped from our care. I wanted the world to know how horrible they all were—our agency, DSS, and the girls' attorney. They were all in on it together, aligned for the common goal of boosting the percentages of their reunification program. Ignoring therapist's recommendations and retraumatizing the children they were supposed to be protecting. And they had made us seem like the ones who were wrong, like we were crazy for caring and advocating for their sanity. A month later and all the veiled and not-so-veiled implications of their rhetoric still stung. I so wanted to cuss them all out. I wanted to tell them all that they could rot in hell. But I was sick and weary of fighting. They would never understand the significance of what I was saying, as they were already so devoid of human emotion or care. These people were numb to the pain they were promoting for the kids unlucky enough to be part of the system. A system they were all too proud to have created. So I gave it to God, waiting, believing, and hoping that someday he would make it right. I still kept in touch with the girls' step grandmother, and it was a relief when I found out the girls were in fact OK. They had asked about us though. I could only imagine what they had been told. I hoped they'd never believe that we didn't want them.

Speaking of stinging, my IVF injections had increased to three shots a day, all in my belly. Of course, it lined up directly with our vacation to Florida, so we had to travel with the bag full of various medications and syringes. Like the visual learner I am, I had taken videos of the nurse putting together the correct needles with each medication. I acted like I understood what she was doing even though I hadn't the slightest idea, nor was I processing it. Thankfully, this was Aaron's area of expertise. Even though he nervously studied the videos, watching them repeatedly, he was an expert at administering the injections with precision. I became more appreciative of this skill as the daily regimen of dosages increased and decreased based on the results of my blood work. The most frustrating thing aside from the pinching, bruising, and hormonal side effects was keeping track of all the medications. I tend to be organized in my disorganization, but I could not get a handle on this, and traveling out of state and back again didn't help anything. When we got to Florida and started the addition of the two injections Gonal and Menopur, we realized I hadn't brought the right needle to go with the Menopur. Silly me, I had only brought three different kinds, none of which could inject the right dosage in the way that was needed for that injection. Thankfully, Aaron ran out to Walgreens and saved the day.

The first night we were back in town, even though both of us had checked the suitcase prior to leaving, the Lupron went missing. We freaked out, frantically searched the house, and called two pharmacies in a panic, who did not carry the medication because it had to be sent via a specialty pharmacy. Just when I was at the peak of my freak-out, with the negative thought that maybe I was just not meant to have kids playing over and over in my mind, I decided to search Aaron's bag one more time. And buried way beneath his slacks was the little bottle of Lupron. Thank God! I did not want to have to do this process all over again from the beginning. Stupid, little, fuckin' medication bottle. Ugh. Now that the panic had dissipated and we were relieved from finding the bottle, Aaron began the intricate process of my nightly injections. My

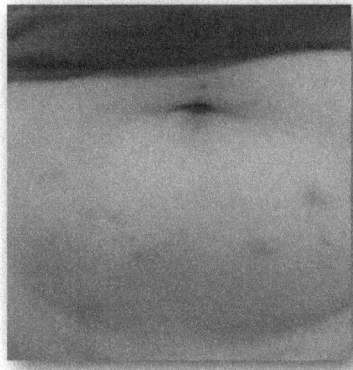
My bruised belly

poor stomach was starting to look like a sad imitation of a rainbow with all the little bruised spots from the injections. Tonight, my belly decided to be extremely uncooperative, and it was like the needle had hit a brick wall. My stomach was almost refusing to take the injection, so Aaron really had to push it in there. Yikes, burning, bleeding pain. This had to lead to something positive, like a healthy baby or five, right? That's what I kept telling myself.

The week of the stimulation process prior to the egg retrieval was probably the most difficult. I was getting three different daily injections along with having to take a vitamin-D pill weekly and a prenatal vitamin daily. Along with that, I had to get blood work every two days to measure my estrogen levels. As I shared earlier, my veins can be more reluctant to come out of hiding than the groundhog when there are six weeks left of winter, so I had one vein that kept being the go-to for drawing blood. My poor vein. It was a weird, draining routine, figuratively and literally: get blood taken around seven o'clock in the morning with an ultrasound here and there, because nothing says good morning like a speculum up your hoo-ha and a needle in your arm; go to work rocking a bandage as an accessory; call for my blood work results; work all day; and then greet my husband, only to have him diligently mix together my nightly injections. Not forgetting the fun game of "how's my stomach going to react tonight?" Will it bleed, burn, reject the injection, or all three? I don't know who it hurt worse, me physically or Aaron emotionally. His hand became shakier each night, as he did not want to hurt me in any way.

It really got fun on the weekend. Not only did I get to wake up early on Saturday morning for blood work and an ultrasound but I also got to do that Sunday morning. On Sunday, Aaron got to see the sonogram, which was pretty exciting. My follicles looked really good, as I was over fifteen at that point. They were measuring the eggs inside the follicles to ensure they had reached the proper size for retrieval, and boy, had they? Finally, my body was cooperating, at least on the inside. Then, it occurred to me that this might actually really take well, and we could end up with quadruplets. But that excited me more than terrified me after everything we had been through.

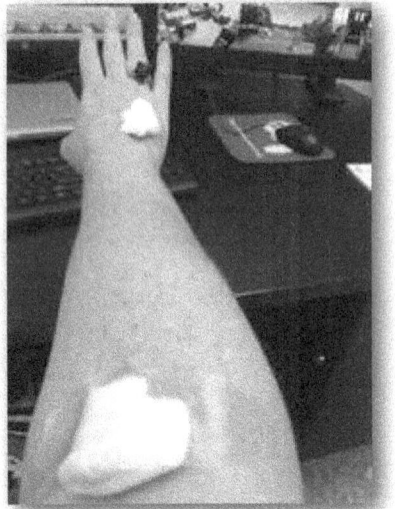

Me rocking my bandages like they're accessories

The nurse explained how to administer the trigger shot that night, worrying Aaron even more, because he would have to give it to me in the upper quadrant of my posterior. There were always so many steps that were explained. I nodded my head, attempting to listen, but when it got into these drawn-out medication steps, I zoned out almost immediately. Thankfully, Aaron was hanging on every word and asked the annoyed doctor if he could take a video, which she let him do as long as her face was not in it. When I called later to check on the results of my blood work, I was told the exact time we needed to do the trigger-shot injection: 9:00 p.m. The egg retrieval would be on Tuesday. I knew the date finally. We were progressing. Aaron would have to start prepping at 8:30 p.m.

Of course, when magic time came, it was not as easy as the doctor made it seem. He had to get the needle in without drawing blood, so first he had to ensure it was just air and bubbles. He barely stuck it in on the "X marks the spot" of my butt before blood came spurting out and running down my cheek. At this point, he was freaking out, so I had to remain calm to get him stabilized, as we couldn't let minutes tick by. He frantically ran and got another needle, and we attempted round two. This time, I craned my neck around, trying to point to the X while also looking in the mirror simultaneously. Of course, a part of the problem was that Aaron had lost his glasses while we were on vacation and had not yet gotten them replaced, so his eyesight was failing him. But it wasn't the time or the place to nag about that, even though I wanted to. After all, I was the one being drilled in the rear repeatedly with a needle. Shouldn't I be the one freaking out from the blood that had now gushed all the way down my leg? But no, I remained calm. There's that assistant principal in me remaining cool, calm, and collected in an emergency situation. "You got this, honey," I said in my most steady, confident voice. Take two: needle in. Air and bubbles, check. Long needle inserted. Ouch. Needle out and more gushing blood. Whew, it was done. However, my ass hurt so bad that I could hardly lie on that side for the rest of the night.

The next morning I awoke earlier than my alarm. I felt at peace, happy even, with a spring in my step that had been notably missing since we lost the girls. I fed the animals, did the dishes, made my lunch, sipped my tea, and was out the door for my now-routine date with the fertility center for more blood work, as well as an ultrasound. Although I had immediately started drinking water when I woke up, my vein decided it had had enough! My poor little surface vein on my right arm sputtered out a couple of droplets of blood and then quit producing it, pushing the needle out. So the doctor had to use the vein in my hand, which hurt more but worked effectively. Eh, what's one more bandage and bruise at this point? She then talked me through the procedure that would occur the next day, having me sign the necessary forms and reviewing my health history. This was going to be another surgical procedure, but after the last stint in the hospital, I felt like I knew what to expect with the health-history forms and anesthesia process, so all the jabber about consent did not make me as nervous as it had during the last round.

Then, it was off to the ultrasound. Today, I got to see my actual doctor. Hello, cold gel, and the speculum was in. She probed around as usual. It was a lot more uncomfortable then before. She explained that it would be due to the size of my ovaries at that point. She was pleased at the amount of follicles on my right side. At this point, I was taking praise about my ovaries like I had just won the Miss America Pageant, beaming proudly every time they were given a compliment. She went to print out the first sonogram picture. Nothing. She fiddled around, thinking out loud: "The printer is offline? What does that mean?" She called in the other doctor. They both fiddled around with wires. The whole time, the speculum was still inside of me. Yet another doctor came in. She finally took the speculum out. My growing discomfort was overcome by her frustration with the machine and the technology. At this point she was saying, "Jesus Marian Joseph," and other things that all involved Jesus. It was hilarious! If I didn't laugh about it in my mind, I would actually absorb the pain and want to cry, thinking, *Woe is me*, because earlier in the week, I had been in the same awkward position, when the sonogram ran out of printer paper. This sonogram definitely had it in for me. But at this point there was no time to wonder why certain things always seemed to happen. This was happening! It was going positive, and tomorrow was the day my future baby could be mixed up in a test tube. Even though my arm looked ridiculous with the multiple bandages and my body was bruised, my spirit felt like a conqueror.

On the morning of the procedure, I woke up more excited than nervous. I was anxiously ready to reap the harvest of the massive amount of medication torture I had been putting my body through. Since things had gone so smoothly, I was confident that, with the number of follicles, we would get a good number of eggs. My mom and Aaron accompanied me to the procedure. Once we got there, we were all taken back into a hidden operating room. It was right by the registration desk; who knew? I had been coming in almost every day and had no idea it even existed. The standard directions were given regarding undressing and putting on the glamorous gown and shower cap, along with the comfy socks. Because the procedure was in the morning, and this time I was smart with my food and water intake, I was not very uncomfortable with my level of thirst or hunger.

I never feel more popular than when I am awaiting surgery. There is always a line of people to talk to you, explain their role in the procedure, and answer any questions. Like clockwork, I met with the scrub nurse, the anesthesiologist, the embryologist, and my doctor. The embryologist was the person I paid the most attention to, since this process of follicles, eggs, and embryos (are they fertilized, not fertilized, viable, not viable?) was foreign to me. She explained that when they extracted the eggs from the follicles, they

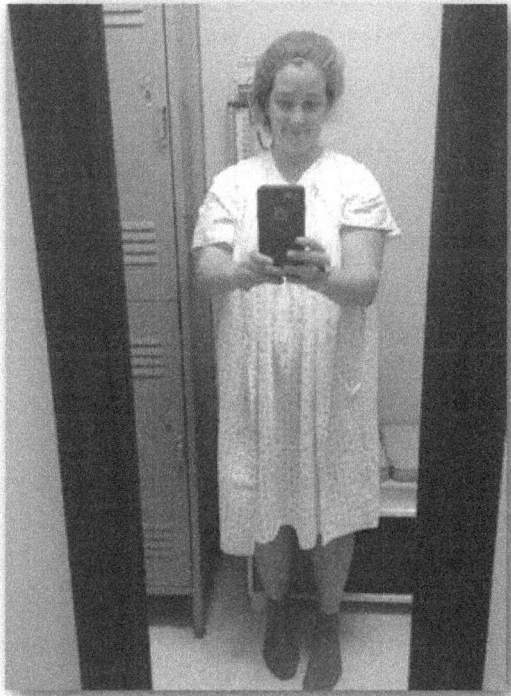

All decked out and ready for the procedure. C'mon, eggs!

would examine them to see which ones were mature, which meant unbroken. The immature, unbroken ones would never be used. Then she would monitor them to see how they were fertilizing with the sperm. The minimum goal would be to get three embryos for the blastocyst. I find *blastocyst* to be such an interesting name. It really does represent everything you are hoping for in IVF: the embryos being in the best fertilized state, which means it is ideal to wait for five days to determine which ones are viable to then blast off to the uterus. That's my definition, not Wikipedia's. Anyway, I really didn't know or care too much about the blastocyst until I was getting this lengthy explanation. This was the goal, because there was more success this way. Got it! Come on, follicles; do your thing and produce some good-quality, mature eggs!

It wasn't long until I was ready to be wheeled in on the gurney. Although Aaron was supposed to go to the work, at that point I could tell his stress level had hit maximum, so I told him it would be fine to call out. At that point, I couldn't imagine not being by his side after the procedure. He was my rock. They wheeled me into the cold room. As I looked up, I noticed they had wall decals filled with flowers, butterflies, hearts, and inspirational words like *faith* to look at. How reassuring! I complimented them, took a deep sigh, and listened as the anesthesiologist explained the effect that the medication was about to have on me. I was well aware of anesthesia and certainly ready for it, as I did not want to be awake for them extricating follicles out of my ovaries. Not a sight I needed to see. And that was it; my mind was blank, not asleep, not high, just a blank space of nothing until the procedure had concluded.

I've had anesthesia before, and although the recovery process has been quite weird and interesting, it has never been as uncomfortable and disorienting as it was that day. Even though they told me they were going to get me conscious in the recovery room, I was not prepared to be so startled. It felt like I was younger and my mom was telling me to wake up for school. I kept opening my eyes, but all I wanted to do was shut them immediately again and drift back into a blank state. When I did finally get them open, I somehow managed to get myself off the operating table and onto the gurney as they directed. I was very groggy. I was then able to lie on the bed in the recovery/

preoperation area. They told me it went very well, and they were able to get eleven follicles. Great! I asked for Aaron, knowing that he had taken off work. They told me that it was just my mom in the waiting room, because he had gone home to get the house ready for me. I tried to tell myself my mom being there would be enough, that Aaron was helping me by being home, but all I wanted was to see his face, have him beside me, and feel the comfort that only his presence provided when I was at my weakest.

As they sat me up and gave me some water to sip, my mom was brought back. She told me how well it went and repeated the follicle number. I asked about Aaron, and as I was listening to her respond, I started to feel extremely weird: dizzy, like I was going to pass out, and sick. I heard a dinging sound behind me, alerting all who were within the vicinity that something was clearly wrong. The staff came rushing over, sat me back, gave me something in my IV, and put a breathing tube in. To say this was unsettling was putting it mildly. I felt so disoriented and afraid. My body had never reacted like this after coming off anesthesia! Ugh. Thank God one of my talents is working with kids on calming them down, so I took a page out of those techniques and just tried to breathe. Good thing I hadn't been able to see myself, because I was told that my fingernails had turned purple and my lips blue before I was finally at a stable, consistent heart rate. It figures this would happen when Aaron wasn't there.

After twenty minutes of additional recovery time, I was able to get dressed to go home. They told me to rest for the remainder of the day and that I could resume "normal" activities the next day. I was also told to call to check on my eggs the next morning at eight o'clock. Even though I was in pain, I was excitedly waiting to hear how my embryos were going to do. The number eleven had to mean a great outcome. At least, I was naive enough to think that, only having a limited understanding of embryo development. Aaron had called on our way out the door to talk to my mom. He must have sensed that something was wrong, because he had gotten in the car and started driving to the fertility center when he didn't hear from us. I checked my purse. Yup, I missed his call. Too busy turning blue to have answered, honey. The rest of the day was a groggy, sore blur. After I got in bed, ate, and watched a TV show, I passed out and was in and out of sleep. It hurt to turn certain ways, and the pressure in my belly along with the full feeling felt identical to after my myomectomy. Every time I stood or sat, it was excruciating. When I found myself coherent, all I could think about were my embryos. I hoped they were doing well. I never thought I would be so excited to call and discuss the status of eggs.

The next morning, still in pain but having to go to work, as I was the only one who could cover the office that day, I got up early, anticipating being in my office for the "egg status" phone call. I went about my normal morning routine and was getting something in the basement when my husband told me I had just missed a call. It wasn't even eight o'clock yet. Hmm. He called right back, and I was directly on the line with the embryologist, who launched into the status of the embryos. Out of the eleven eggs, only seven were mature. Four were viable, but one became abnormal. So out of all eleven, only three had made it to the next level, and it was only eight o'clock in the morning on the day after the procedure. I felt like I was a hot-air balloon that someone had just shot. My heart sank, my excited demeanor deflated, and I hunched over. I heard myself saying, "So that's not good, right?" Aaron rushed to sit next to me, putting his arm around me simultaneously. The embryologist went into full detail about the process of abnormalities and the state of the embryos, emphasizing that we would only need three, but exactly three, for the blastocyst. I was to call the next day at eleven o'clock to check on the status from there.

To say that I was devastated would be an understatement. I felt my emotions rising up inside me, my thoughts revolving around negativity, telling me that they weren't going to make it and that I had put myself through all this pain for nothing. When I get like that, I just need to get away from people, shut up, and try to get my head right. Good thing I had to go manage my office. Aaron knew how much pain I was in and mustered something along the lines of "Keep the faith and be positive." I love him, but not good timing. I immediately snapped at him that it wasn't his body that was going through all of this, stormed off, and drove emotion riddled on the way to work. At this point I was so late that it was no surprise I got stopped behind a school bus and had no choice but to wait an extra fifteen minutes. Along with getting frustrated when I get stuck in a traffic jam I didn't anticipate, I often find myself getting introspective. The flashing, immovable bus was so comparable to the situation in my life: a roadblock I had no control over preventing me from getting to the destination I wanted to go to.

Thankfully, all my years in education have taught me how to go into my teacher smile, masking whatever inner turmoil I'm experiencing. I was also appreciative that it was the summer, there was no summer school, and inter-actions with people would be minimal. When I saw a call pop up from the doctor's office at around eleven o'clock, I knew the news was not going to be positive. It was the embryologist. When she just went to check on the three remaining embryos, one was developing abnormally chromosome-wise, so it had to be discarded. This meant the blastocyst at day five was no longer an option. She explained that we would do the embryo transfer with the remain-ing two the next day. Inside, I hoped they would make it to the next day. I hung up the phone, and immediately the office phone started ringing. It was a lady in the community wanting to know when the grass behind the school would be mowed. *Fucking seriously?* I thought. However, being the trained professional I am, I responded with polite respect and gave her the informa-tion for the program associated with that, which is not through my school system.

"So do you know which department I should start with?" she persisted.

Breathe, Chrissie, just breathe. In the most pleasant sing-song voice I could muster, I told her I did not. This is the call I get after the devastating embryo update? Really? I regrouped; then I texted our community substitute, who was a godsend, to see if she could cover the office, filling her in on the situa-tion. She always came through whenever needed. Especially in an upsetting time like this one, I was more and more appreciative for people like that in my life. That year, the people at my school had really become my family, going through each up and down with me while I attempted to foster to adopt.

The rest of the day I was drowning in my feelings, so after sending a prayer request to Joyce Meyer, I googled some information on day-two embryo transfers, looking at only the positive blogs. Most of the ones I read had moms who were pregnant as a result. In addition, with an embryo transfer, there is a greater chance of twins. That would be amazing! Even though my emotions were sinking, I tried to force my mind to be positive. I didn't exactly win the battle, but I at least kept my mouth shut, not letting out negative thoughts for the remainder of the day. This emotional roller coaster just kept perplexing me. Throughout our entire journey so far, it had started positive, and then the bottom had dropped out from under us just when we felt like we were moving in a hopeful direction. How much more of this could I take? I didn't know if I could endure the pain of the IVF process again, and it was something I prayed I wouldn't have to go through. Because, damn it, these were our two strongest embryos. They were going to make it. I was impossible, right? The doctors told my mom she wouldn't carry me to term even after lying on one side for eight weeks. When I was born prematurely, I wasn't going to make it without a heart transplant. Well, I did. That was what my blood was about. Our baby was going to happen. All we needed was one! As I drifted off into an unrestful sleep, those were the thoughts I was trying to focus on to squash the negative ones trying to bubble up.

I awoke the next day renewed with positivity and feeling refreshed. Aaron had taken off for the day, thank God. I couldn't go through another procedure without him there the whole time. Since I read that it was good to have activity instead of rest after the transfer, we made a plan to have a date day after the procedure and to go out to lunch as well as a funny movie in our favorite theater where there was reserved seating.

We got to the fertility center early. My mom also met us there. She was super excited to be a part of things. It was a good thing we did get there early, because, of course, I had not brought the medicine I was supposed to. I swear, keeping track of these medications—when to take what, how to administer it, and the dosage—was more complicated than calculus for me. Aaron, being the dutiful, supportive man that he is, immediately ran home to get the medication. It wasn't long until we were taken back, my blood was drawn for the millionth time, and the nurse administered my shot. Of course, I got scolded because I had somehow missed that I was supposed to have Aaron give me this butt shot with the oil the day before. Luckily, she was able to administer a double dose. Whew! Again, it was gown time, and this time I would have a family audience for the embryo transfer. Even though it was my mom and Aaron, it's still always uncomfortable having multiple people watch as you get things inserted up your hoo-ha. I was supposed to come with a half-full bladder. Remembering the nightmare of an overly full bladder at my first sonogram, I did my best to comply. My bladder always felt full anyway. I explained this to the nurse, but wouldn't you know it, the one time I needed the damn thing to be full, it was not at the right capacity. So I had to down a bottle of water. After twenty minutes, they checked again. Nope, still not there. Another bottle of water. At this point, I felt like I could float away.

Finally, after forty minutes and three checks on the sonogram machine, we were ready to go. I had no idea what to expect, but with the nurse, the doctor, Aaron, my mom, and me, there certainly was a captive audience. The doctor explained every step as he went, which I appreciated. Slide down, the speculum went in. Ugh, uncomfortable but not painful. No cramping, nope, just awkward. Then they slid a tube above to transport the embryos. I had my head turned toward Aaron and was holding his hand as he and my mom watched the tube slide into my uterus on the sonogram machine, depositing our two strong embryos, one of which we had now nicknamed Pokey. I squeezed his hand harder as the discomfort got stronger. It felt like a preview of things to come when I would be delivering our long-awaited baby.

When the procedure was completed, they checked the tube to ensure the embryos had in fact deposited. They confirmed they had and explained how smoothly they went. I was very thankful. God, I wanted this to work. I didn't know if I could go through this process again. We had a wonderful day after that and remained extremely positive. I only had two more blood tests to go before the waiting ensued for the pregnancy test. For the blood tests, they were checking my estrogen levels. I had stopped having to have the butt shot full of progesterone oil and was now on a good-morning daily insert of estrogen up my vagina. This was almost a relief at this point after having to get shot after shot for the past month. My estrogen levels were good, and no additional hormone was needed. Feeling as if I knew my body, I thought the difficult part for us had always been getting the egg fertilized and into the right area. Now that that portion was done, I felt strongly like my body would take over and naturally do what I knew it could do. I read everything I could about embryo implantation.

For the next week and a half, my body started doing some strange things. I felt cramping for several days on one side. I hoped that was Pokey implanting himself. It was very weird cramping and unlike any I had ever experienced before. One night, as I got up from bed, there was a very strong smell of what I guessed was something tomato based with a hint of cat throw-up. I asked Aaron if he was cooking anything in the microwave, and he said SpaghettiOs. Well, who in the hell smells SpaghettiOs? That had to be a good sign, right? Several days later, I also smelled the strong odor of mouse urine in my office. That made sense, because there was a mouse family there that had been vying for my job as assistant principal with the amount of time they were spending on my desk. My custodian had battled them, putting down multiple mouse traps until they were caught. And my breasts. *Oh my God!* They were so heavy and full. Not to mention the fact that I had this strange, tingling, burning feeling in my nipples. They were so painful that the one day I tried to wear a bra, I literally felt like I had heartburn in my boobs and I was going to die. I discreetly took my bra off midafternoon and hadn't worn one since. At night, the only relief I got was from Icy Hot patches on them and hot showers. My boobs felt like they weighed twenty pounds. Could this all mean pregnancy, or was I manufacturing these symptoms in my mind? The other thing I wondered was if it was all just side effects from the hormones being inserted into my body on a daily basis.

Food was also starting to taste different. Normally, I would drink fruit smoothies in the morning and/or ginger ale or seltzer water. I wanted none of that. The only things I liked seemed to be strawberry Snapple and lemonade. And I only wanted either salads with turkey or fruit or creamy things like alfredo, white pizza, and cream cheese. I also had a queasy yet starving feeling at different points during the day that would manifest as crankiness, and I could kill someone at any minute if I didn't get something to eat. When I would get my food, again, if anyone touched it or interrupted me, I felt like I could murder him or her. Lucky Aaron, right?

Everything that I read said this wait would be the hardest part of the IVF process. I was scaring myself, because I felt so positive that I was pregnant. My body was being very weird, and yet at the same time, I had difficulty imagining the nurse actually saying the words, "You're pregnant." This had been the Holy Grail for so long, the unattainable dream for four years. I was so used to the news going in a positive direction and then being dropped out from under me that I couldn't imagine it going in a different direction. Aaron and I had decided in this waiting period that if the news was negative, we would try again with IVF. Now all we had to do was wait until the twenty-fifth. I shouldn't have, but I started looking up baby decor and maternity wear. I felt pregnant. I also couldn't shake the timing of everything. I believe God has a purpose for everything—the cliché that everything happens for a reason. Had the embryos made it to day five, our timetable would not have happened the way it did. As it happened, I had my embryo transfer two days before what would have been my grandma's ninety-seventh birthday, and we were finding out we were pregnant the day of the girls' court case. The date that had been etched in my mind for the past five months. I just knew there had to be a reason for all of it. Like all the pain and heartbreak we had gone through would be overturned into a positive miracle on that date if we found out we were pregnant and the girls were able to go home to their grandparents, in turn leading to us being able to be a part of their lives again. And wouldn't it be exciting if the next time I saw them I could tell them we were expecting? Almost the whole time we had them, they had wanted us to have a baby. The little one had even named the baby. She proclaimed that the baby's name would be Cody, Cody Kahan. I actually rather liked it.

The weekend before we found out the news, we stumbled onto the movie *Southpaw* that Saturday evening. What a phenomenal movie! However, the portrayal of the childcare system was laughable considering our personal experiences. At one point the caseworker says to him that he is too much of a mess to see his daughter. Yeah right, like they would ever prevent a biological parent from seeing the child, let alone actively supervise and intervene if needed. This is the problem with foster-care portrayals in movies. They make you think that the state makes it difficult for biological parents to get their kids back when actually the state does everything in its power to get the kids back with their biological parents, all because their "research" and "percentages," which they skew, say that is in the best interest of the child. Forget the behaviors the kids display, because even though it is a case-by-case basis for most things, *all* foster-care kids display behaviors, so it is no big deal.

The day before we found out, I had my worst bouts of fear, negativity, and anxiety. I almost didn't want to know. For so long we had hoped, tried, and waited, with the end result never being what we wanted. This felt different. I certainly felt pregnant, but what if my body was playing tricks on me? What if it was all my mind and my hormones manifesting these symptoms? Before I knew it, tears were streaming down my face at the fear of negative news. It was a long day, but Aaron and I talked it out, taking comfort in the fact that we were feeling the same way. We knew, no matter what the news was, we would get through it together. That night I did my best to sleep and to try to remain positive. My body and mind were telling me I was pregnant. I was just petrified that the actual test wouldn't confirm it. So I did what I had learned over the years to calm my mind and focused on scripture. The following scripture came into my mind: "Trust in the Lord with all your heart and lean not on your own understanding: In all your ways acknowledge him and he shall direct your paths." That, along with the ocean-sound app on my phone, finally lulled me to sleep. I had found a really cute meme with the *Game of Thrones* Stark symbol in the womb announcing that "Baby is Coming." I hoped I would get to use it to tell Aaron the next day.

Today was the day. I was positive and hopeful. Surely, my body couldn't be lying to me this time. I had been home from work that morning, as we were getting work done on our house. The girls' departure had been a catalyst, and we decided that we were finally going to make our dream of moving to Florida happen within the next year, which meant getting the house ready to sell. The night before, I had dreamed that the girls were back with us, except this time we had a baby. That had to be a good sign.

About an hour before I was set to find out, I was getting ready to go to work when my refrigerator started smoking. Quickly the kitchen started becoming engulfed in smoke with a dangerous, chemical smell. I unplugged it and called my boss. No work for me that day. Instead, in the midst of what was supposed to be an exciting day, I would be calling emergency repair services. Then, I got a text from the girls' grandparents. They were not returned. Instead, the system was dragging it out until their next hearing in October. The grandparents would get transitional visits, which meant longer and more frequent visits with the potential of being overnight. My heart broke for all of them. The girls would have to start yet another new school. Then I called the office. I knew immediately by the somber tone of my favorite nurse's voice: "Christine, I'm so sorry to tell you this, but you're not pregnant." I immediately felt the hot tears streaming down my face as she talked about next steps. Within an hour, my hopes along with the refrigerator had literally gone up in smoke. After I let everyone who was praying for my pregnancy know the result, I shut down. After the sadness and tears, I slumped into the familiarity of the numbness. Just like every other experience throughout this journey, it had started with excitement, followed by hope and difficulties, and then every positive hope we had being dropped out from under us. All the shots, all the medication, all the blood work, missing my youth-group trip, not drinking, giving up coffee, for what? Absolutely nothing.

CHAPTER 9

Over the Infertility Rainbow

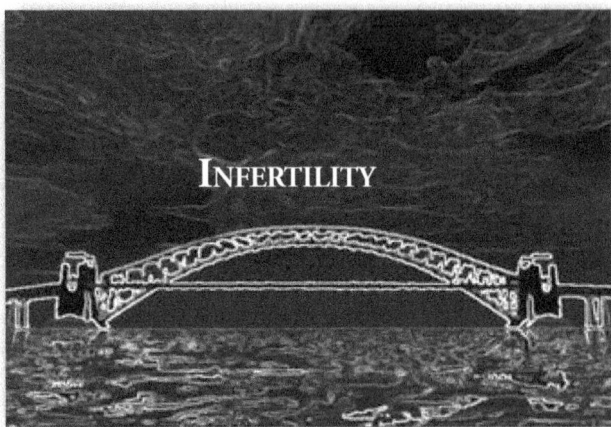

INFERTILITY

July 2016

WHAT NOW? ANOTHER ROUND OF IVF that would probably fail? International adoption? When I looked up the resources I was given for international adoption, my stomach started to churn as I read about the process. I didn't know if I could go through another home study or if I could have my baby dreams dictated by someone else's rules and stipulations. But the more I thought about it, the more I realized they always had been since we set foot down the path of infertility road. My heart ached for the baby I'd thought we had and didn't, but also for the girls. Had they just been able to return to their grandparents, I may have been able to accept the heartbreaking news of not being pregnant with a more positive resolve. Instead, they would be stuck now with this foster family who wasn't taking them to therapy and wasn't keeping up with visits until October. They would have to start *another* new school. The little one was going into kindergarten. I hated that I wouldn't be there for her. That we didn't even have a chance of seeing them until the end of October. I wondered if they were OK and what they were thinking, let alone really feeling. Were they thinking of us? Had their time with us made the impact I thought, or were we just two more people they stayed with for a short time in their lives? My heart just ached. I spent the rest of the day wallowing in my numbness. Aaron came home early, and we went to work out and swim. I amazed even myself at my capacity to continue going on after each disappointment. I don't know why I thought this time it would be different. I let myself be knocked down that day in order to regroup.

Two days later, I got my period. Another red brick. I dutifully called my doctor and started my next round of birth-control pills. I would go through one more round of IVF. This time, since they knew the difficulty my body had, they were going to take a different approach. They were confident it would be successful. I was determined to do everything I could to ensure I had healthy eggs, but I also set my mind to not get too hopeful or excited. As much as I admire those people who continue through three or four rounds of IVF, this would be it for me with this option. After this, Aaron and I would have to explore international adoption. Who knows maybe that is and has been the plan all along. I didn't feel it in my heart quite yet. As I flipped through my phone, I stumbled onto the pictures I had tried so hard to avoid and yet could never delete. My little one at the pool, eating Cheetos, jumping in the water, and having the time of her life. It was the last weekend I spent with her. I missed those girls so much. I had just numbed myself from the pain, but it came back in a wave, and before I knew it, there were tears welling up in my eyes. It felt like the grieving process of a death: denial, anger, depression, bargaining, and acceptance.

If this were a movie or a thirty-minute sitcom, everything would be wrapped up happily. We would be pregnant with twins, and the girls would somehow be back in our lives. We would be one big happy family, with the turmoil we've suffered in our rearview mirror. However, this is real life, and as much as I wanted a happy ending for this story, I don't have one. I wish that I could tell you that the pain, the procedures, the processes we went through led to our dreams of becoming parents. But it hasn't. What it has done is tested our marriage, tested my faith, and led me up and down throughout a roller coaster of emotions. As I write this, we continue with our second round of IVF. We continue with our prayers for the two little girls we loved, who are stuck in another foster home in a system that is refusing to relinquish them back to the family they knew for two years and who love them more than anything.

A lot of people have said to me that they didn't know I had been through all of this and continue going. As I was trying to find a way to give this story a worthy written ending, I came across a video on social media articulating a lesson a father was trying to teach his daughter, who had determined she could no longer face the obstacles in life because they just kept coming one after another. He boiled three pots of water, putting in potatoes, eggs, and coffee. When they were done, the potatoes had gone from hard to soft, the eggs had gone from fragile to hardened, and yet the coffee remained unchanged by the water. The father explained that in spite of each of these items facing the same obstacle, the coffee was the only one that had not changed. Instead, the coffee was the one that changed the water and made it into something new. The father asked the girl which one she would be. I already know which one I am. I am without a doubt the coffee, which is why I wanted to get this story out. Because these experiences will not harden me. In turn, they will also not break me down into someone soft who would easily sacrifice his or her beliefs. Instead, I am hoping that if enough people read this, they will know that we all can be the coffee, changing the water together.

No goal or dream in my life has ever been easily obtained. God has always taken me on a difficult road through a lot of pain. I have never known the meaning of the pain in that time, but later on God will use it for me to help someone else. My hope is just that overarching purpose. For all of you out there who are struggling with infertility, *you* are not alone! For those of you who have loved and lost a child in the foster-care system, a child you wanted to give a permanent home, *you* are not alone! And if there is anyone out there who has had a negative experience with that system because you loved and advocated for children even when everyone in the system told you to back down, I stand with you.

If anyone reading this book can help, I am begging you, as there are two little girls whom I love more than anything in this world being forced to stay in a system that they do not deserve, all because a dictator in charge has deemed that it is in their "best interest" and promotes a program where "reunification" is the way. She believes this above everything else, no matter the retraumatization to the child or children involved. We have a country right now that has condoned having people take a drug test to keep their welfare, but in most states, they can be convicted of abuse or murder, have a drug addiction, and utterly neglect their children and still ultimately almost always get their children back. That will never make sense to me. And to those of you reading this who never had a similar experience, I hope that my journey has opened your eyes to the thoughts and pain that those of us with infertility struggle with in trying to achieve the blessing of being parents, which is supposed to be a natural rite of passage.

But then again, I'm infertile. I'm so far down my journey of infertility that there is no way back. Any child to me would be a sacred gift I would like to think I would cherish forever. However, no matter what, I keep going, putting one foot in front of the other, being that coffee, sometimes bitter, sometimes with two sugars and cream, because I still have 575 kids I can watch over, advocate for, and be a positive influence for. And at the end of the day, that makes me very blessed! If our story helps even one person out there, it will have been worth it. Never give up on your dreams, even if you are having difficulty navigating the road of infertility.

Do you have a personal story to share? If so, log onto http://www.kingkahan. com/ and subscribe. Chrissie or Aaron will send you a personalized message in return.

www.ingramcontent.com/pod-product-compliance
Lightning Source LLC
Chambersburg PA
CBHW030014290326
41934CB00005B/332